The Poison in Your Teeth

The Poison in Your Teeth

Mercury Amalgam (Silver) Fillings . . .
Hazardous to Your Health!

Tom McGuire, DDS

The Dental Wellness Institute
SEBASTOPOL

Lead Editor: Kristi Lanier
Assistant Editor: Zoe Rivers
Assistant Editor: Sylvia Wallach
Cover Design: Buffie Harris/Lynda Banks
Indexer: Sheila M. Ryan
eBook Consultant: Kevin Bjornsen
Website Adaptation: Marty Roberts

Library of Congress Catalog Card Number: 2008901675
ISBN 978-0-9815630-0-8

9 8 7 6 5 4 3 2 1

To my wife, Zoe.

Without your love and support this book would not have been written.

Thank you for the sacrifices you've made and for being such

a wonderful friend. I love you!

Disclaimer

The material in this book is for information purposes only. It does not make any medical, dental, or special claims. Neither does it attempt to diagnose or treat any ailment, dental or medical. It does not encourage self-diagnosis or self-treatment. Nor is it intended to be, and should not be, used as a replacement for appropriate treatment by a qualified dentist, physician, or other health professional. The publisher and author do not assume liability or responsibility for any injury, damage, or loss alleged to be caused by the use, effectiveness, or safety of any suggestions, procedures, or products mentioned in this book. The reader must take full responsibility for verifying any personal observations through consultation with a licensed dentist, dental hygienist, or qualified health professional.

The publisher and author have made every effort to ensure the completeness and accuracy of the information presented in this book. The publisher and author cannot be held responsible for any inadvertent errors or omissions, or for how this information is interpreted and/or applied. The author has made a sincere effort to ensure that Internet addresses and other contact information were accurate at the time this book was published. We cannot assume responsibility for those that changed after publication.

Contents

List of Tables

Acknowledgements

So many people contributed to this book, and through them I've learned that no author stands alone. Space doesn't allow me to thank everyone who helped make this book possible, so if I leave anyone out, I apologize.

Many thanks to Kristi Lanier, a very special editor and writer. My gratitude to Buffie Harris and Lynda Banks, both very talented artists and graphic designers, who worked together to create the book's cover. I'm deeply thankful to Sylvia Wallach and Zoe Rivers, who did a great job with the initial editing and contributed so much to making sure that what I wrote would be understood. Kevin Bjornsen, a computer genius and friend, is responsible for the eBook version. Many thanks to Oriana Leckert, an extraordinarily gifted proofreader. No book worth its salt would be all it can be without an indexer—thank you, Sheila M. Ryan. I want to thank Roberta Ryan, business coach extraordinaire, for all of her help and organizational genius, and Marsha Sendar, a gifted nutrition consultant who was kind enough to share her wisdom.

I also want to acknowledge some very special people who, in their own way, supported me during the times I needed support, whether they knew it or not: Gertrude and David Mablin, Roger Squire, Dennis and Claire Noble, Sacha Mons, Stefanie Wallach, Onie Kriegler, Steve Guerra and Leslie Johnson, Joan Faxon, Steve Foster, Paul and Nancy Rubin, Marty Roberts, Phil Green, Beau Connell, Virginia Bell, Jerry and Kathy Colletto, and Dawn, Christina, and Mikayla Owen. My special thanks to Chris Hall.

Everyone I've mentioned is special to me, and this book wouldn't be what it is without their help.

Foreword

As a mercury free and mercury safe holistic dentist, I am constantly looking for new insights into the subject of mercury amalgam (silver) fillings. I am particularly interested in accessing information about this topic that is accurate and easy to understand. I do this not only for my own personal knowledge, but also because I believe I have a responsibility to my patients. And that responsibility is to make sure I provide them with the best information on this subject so they can make informed decisions about their dental treatment.

The controversy surrounding the health hazards of mercury amalgam fillings is still raging, and while progress has been made, it may be years before they're banned in the U.S. When Dr. Tom McGuire asked me to write the Foreword to his book, *The Poison in Your Teeth: Mercury Amalgam (Silver) Fillings . . . Hazardous to Your Health*, I readily accepted. This book is the first I have read that provides a single source of objective and definitive information and addresses every aspect of this subject. Dr. McGuire's other important books—*Tooth Fitness: Your Guide to Healthy Teeth*; *The Tooth Trip*; and *Mercury Detoxification: The Natural Way to Remove Mercury from Your Body*—are excellent sources of information about oral health.

After reading *The Poison in Your Teeth*, I knew Dr. McGuire had written another winner. Not only is it a factual, informative, and well-documented book, it's also extraordinarily easy to read and understand. Even if you have no prior knowledge of amalgam fillings or chronic mercury poisoning, you will be very well informed by the time you finish reading. The book will take you through every step of the process needed to understand how these toxic fillings can harm your health by releasing highly poisonous mercury vapor into your body. In particular, Chapter 4: "Chronic Mercury Poisoning and Amalgam (Silver) Fillings" provides the best explanation I've found about the cause-and-effect connection between amalgam fillings and mercury.

Mercury vapor released from dental fillings can directly or indirectly contribute to—or make worse—nearly every known disease or health problem. If you have these poisonous fillings and don't take the proper steps to have them safely removed, you may be putting your health at risk.

Some of the important topics discussed in this book are:

- symptoms and diseases related to chronic mercury poisoning

- the health improvements seen when amalgams are safely removed and the mercury is cleared from the body

- the safe removal protocol needed to minimize a patient's exposure to mercury during the amalgam removal process

- mercury free and mercury safe dentists—what they do and how to find one

- mercury detoxification and the importance of safely removing mercury from the body

- healing the damage done by mercury

Dr. McGuire also gives a brief and interesting history of these poisonous fillings and offers his opinion as to why the American Dental Association (ADA) continues to defend them.

Chapter 6: "The Effects of Mercury on the Fetus, Nursing Baby, and Child" deserves particular praise. Here, Dr. McGuire describes how exposure to mercury poisoning from amalgam fillings can occur at the moment of conception, long before the child grows up and has its own amalgam fillings. It categorically connects mercury from amalgam fillings to autism and other learning, mental, and developmental disorders.

The Poison in Your Teeth was written for everyone with these toxic fillings and everyone thinking about having them put in. It's a must for women who are planning to have a family. This book is just as important for those who intuitively feel they should have these fillings safely removed but don't understand exactly why, or to what degree, they can harm your health.

The book's audience also includes all mercury safe dentists who want to provide their patients with the credible, third-party information they'll need to make the important decision about having their mercury amalgam fillings safely removed. I strongly encourage every pro-amalgam dentist who is willing to look objectively at this issue, beyond the information they've received from the ADA, to read this book. I also believe this book should be read carefully by physicians and other health care professionals. Here is another area where having the right information is so important to properly help patients optimize their health.

I enthusiastically recommend this book to all my patients and to anyone who has an interest in this subject and wants to do everything possible to improve their overall health and well-being.

—Paul Rubin, DDS, MIAOMT

Dr. Rubin is one of the true pioneers in promoting healthy, biocompatible, and mercury free and safe dentistry. He was one of the first members of the International Academy of Oral Medicine and Toxicology (IAOMT). Dr. Rubin has his Mastership in the Academy and is active in not only promoting mercury free and mercury safe dentistry, but in educating the public about the health hazards of water fluoridation and indiscriminate use of fluoride. He has an active practice in Seattle, Washington. Visit Dr. Rubin on the web at www.drpaulrubin.com, contact him by phone at 206-367-6453, or email info@drpaulrubin.com.

One

The Poison in Your Teeth

No book about mercury amalgam fillings will be accurate or make sense unless you first understand some basic facts:

- Mercury is the most poisonous, non-radioactive, naturally occurring substance on our planet.

- There is *no safe or harmless level* of mercury. Just one atom of mercury is harmful to the body.

- Amalgam fillings continuously release poisonous mercury vapor.

- Any form of stimulation that heats an amalgam filling will increase the release of mercury vapor.

- Amalgam fillings are the single greatest source of mercury exposure.

- The first exposure to mercury from amalgam fillings can occur at the moment of conception.

- Mercury passes through the placenta to the fetus and through breast milk to the nursing baby.

- Chronic mercury poisoning can directly and indirectly contribute to and increase the risk and severity of every known disease and health issue.

Think Mercury!

To make sense of what you'll read in this book, it's important to know that 50 percent of an amalgam filling is *mercury,* and many factors influence and determine the amount released. So, as you read this book, never stop thinking *mercury.* When you read the word "amalgam," think *mercury.* When you read the term "silver fillings," think *mercury* fillings! When you read the word "poisonous" or "toxic," think *mercury*!

Always thinking *mercury* is important because pro-amalgam dentists will never use that word when talking about an amalgam or silver filling. Why? Because they know you'd be concerned if you were aware of the fact that amalgam fillings actually contain and release a poison. I'm still amazed at how many people don't think they have mercury fillings because their dentist refers to them as amalgams or silver fillings.

Amalgam (Silver) Fillings: The Vehicle for Mercury

Amalgam fillings are actually delivery vehicles. They carry mercury and release its toxic vapor into your body. When all is said and done, the fillings themselves aren't directly responsible for the health problems related to chronic mercury poisoning—it's the mercury released from them and stored in your body that's the culprit. In fact, if amalgam fillings didn't release mercury vapor, there wouldn't be a controversy surrounding their use.

A simple visual exercise will help explain what I mean. Imagine a pipeline with a faucet at the end. The pipeline carries mercury and the faucet has direct access to your body. When the faucet is turned on, it releases mercury vapor. The pipeline and faucet are equivalent to an amalgam filling. Obviously, the pipe and the faucet aren't what poisons you; it's the mercury they carry and release.

What You Will Discover in this Book

You'll discover facts about mercury and its relationship to amalgam fillings that will surprise you, such as:

- Mercury can poison every cell in the body and brain.

- Amalgam fillings release mercury—often in amounts far exceeding government regulations—by many common forms of stimulation such as chewing gum and tooth grinding.

- Mercury can devastate the immune system by depleting essential antioxidants.

- The *sum total* of exposure from *all sources* of mercury determines its effect on your health.

- Over 100 symptoms, diseases, and syndromes are directly related to chronic mercury exposure.

As I'll often refer to the immune system, a brief introduction will be useful here. Generally speaking, the immune system protects us against germs, micro-organisms, free radicals, toxins, and poisons. Most people think of the immune system as the white blood cells that circulate in the blood vessels and lymphatic system. Although antioxidants aren't cells, when I refer to the immune system I'm also including the role antioxidants play in protecting our bodies from harmful substances.

Mercury is extraordinarily toxic to the fetus and nursing baby. If you're a mother, expectant, or planning to be one, you'll learn how amalgam fillings:

- Expose the baby to mercury from the moment of conception and throughout nursing.

- Could cause, contribute to, or make worse, every childhood disease, including autism and other developmental and learning disorders.

You'll also discover why the effects of mercury on one's health can vary dramatically from person to person. And you'll see why every factor and variable that determines the amount of mercury vapor released from amalgam fillings must be considered. Some of these factors include how many fillings you have, the size of the fillings, how long you've had them, and if you grind your teeth.

Mercury Free, Mercury Safe

You'll learn about amalgam fillings and their relationship to chronic mercury poisoning, and also the very important differences between mercury free and mercury safe dentists. The term "mercury free" doesn't necessarily mean a dentist is also mercury safe. (Whenever I use the term "mercury safe" in the book, I'm referring to a dentist who is both mercury free and mercury safe.)

You'll be introduced to holistic, biological, alternative, and natural dentists and learn how they differ from pro-amalgam dentists. Additionally, you'll learn how to go about the all-important task of finding a mercury free and mercury safe dentist who can safely remove your amalgam fillings. You'll also discover in Chapter 8: "Safely Removing Mercury Amalgam (Silver) Fillings" how a safe removal protocol will dramatically reduce your exposure to mercury.

While removing the source of mercury is a necessary first step, it's still only the first step. In Chapter 11: "Mercury Detoxification" you'll learn about the importance of mercury detoxification—the next, and even more important, step in eliminating mercury from your body and helping it heal from the damage caused by mercury.

Who Benefits

I wrote *The Poison in Your Teeth* because factual and objective information about this controversial subject isn't easy to find. Unfortunately, much of what is available is incomplete, contradictory, or difficult to understand.

If you're confused, uncertain, skeptical, or curious about whether or not mercury amalgam (silver) fillings pose a risk to your health, then this book for you.

If you're a mother, or plan to be one, and want to do everything you can to protect yourself and your child from exposure to mercury, then this book is definitely for you. Mercury has been implicated in autism and other learning and developmental disorders and I will discuss this relationship in detail.

If you've asked a pro-amalgam dentist to remove your mercury amalgam fillings and he or she says they're safe and harmless, but you're still concerned because you've heard mercury is a poison, then this book will be of interest to you.

If you have any symptoms or health issues that are directly or indirectly related to chronic mercury poisoning, if you truly want to improve your health and well-being, you cannot afford to ignore the effects of this powerful poison on your health. Because mercury is continuously released from amalgam fillings, and enters and is stored in the body, these toxic fillings are the primary cause of chronic mercury poisoning.

Chronic mercury poisoning and its related symptoms occur when small amounts of mercury continuously enter the body and accumulate there over time. There are over 100 symptoms and diseases related to chronic mercury poisoning, including chronic fatigue syndrome, memory loss, heart disease, headaches, autoimmune diseases, tremors, and depression. A full list of symptoms is found in Chapter 5: "Symptoms and Diseases Related to Chronic Mercury Poisoning."

Ultimately, *The Poison in Your Teeth* is for you if you've been unable to find the information you need to make an intelligent decision about safely removing these toxic fillings and replacing them with a safe alternative. (I will use the terms mercury and amalgam interchangeably when discussing these fillings.)

Controversy and Confusion

On one hand, the American Dental Association (ADA) and its pro-amalgam supporters say that mercury fillings are completely safe and harmless. They continue to say they aren't a health hazard even though many studies have proved that they release significant amounts of poisonous mercury vapor from many common forms of filling stimulation, such as brushing and eating.

On the other hand, the World Health Organization (WHO) states that there is no safe level of mercury. The vast majority of the world's scientific community, thousands of mercury safe dentists, and every government regulatory agency recognize that mercury is a powerful poison and must be closely monitored and strictly regulated. In January 2008, Norway and Sweden completely banned the use of mercury amalgams. Denmark followed in April of 2008, and Germany and Austria have banned their use in pregnant women and children up to age 18.

The real issue isn't whether amalgams are structurally sound, easy to use, or inexpensive, it's whether mercury amalgam fillings are hazardous to your health. I ask you to keep that in mind as you read this book. I also ask you to keep in mind that what really matters when you consider the "safety" of these fillings is the fact that they release mercury vapor—and *80 percent of that vapor is inhaled and distributed throughout the body.* Over 150 million people in the U.S. have amalgam fillings, and the WHO states that the average person with these fillings could receive more mercury from them than from food (particularly seafood), air, and water combined!

How can it be possible that mercury released from amalgam fillings is considered safe by the ADA but toxic when released from all other sources? *The Poison in Your Teeth* will answer this question and many more about mercury amalgam fillings. It will provide you with all the information you need to make an informed choice. And it will be logically presented in language you can understand.

Of course, any controversy has two sides. With that in mind, I will also present the main arguments the ADA and its supporters use to defend the continued use of these poison-laced fillings. I will respond to each of their arguments and let you decide who makes the most sense.

Solutions

The Poison in Your Teeth doesn't just identify and discuss problems, it offers solutions. With each chapter you'll not only understand more about how and why these fillings are hazardous to your health, but the steps you can take to have them safely removed and improve your overall health. The key to taking charge of your health is to acquire the information needed to make informed and intelligent decisions.

Chapter 12: "Health Improvements Related to Amalgam Removal and Mercury Detoxification" presents a number of studies showing significant health improvements in thousands who've had their amalgam fillings removed.

Every chapter is supported by sound scientific evidence—not by hearsay, emotion, or unsupported opinion. The extensive reference section gives you access to the same information I used to reach my conclusions. This book is factual and not only offers hope, but choices. It gives you the opportunity to choose health over disease and cease being a victim of these toxic, mercury-emitting fillings.

The Demise of Amalgam Fillings

In a 2007 marketing survey of practicing general dentists in the United States, 52 percent reported they were no longer using mercury amalgam fillings. Some of the dentists surveyed criticized amalgam for its toxicity and tendency to fracture teeth. Others defended its long history and believed amalgam was still a superior material to even the latest generation of composite fillings. But the good news here is that, for the first time in more than 150 years, *over 50 percent of general dentists state they no longer use these toxic fillings.*

This is a significant landmark in the battle to ban these fillings. One of the ADA's most consistent arguments in support of amalgam fillings is that amalgam is a very good filling material. But the tide is turning. Mercury safe dentists are no longer the only ones who believe amalgam is not only toxic, but isn't a good dental filling material. Many rank and file members of the ADA are starting to believe it too and are jumping off the doomed ship called "Amalgam."

What's Next

In Chapter 2: "A Brief History of Mercury Amalgam (Silver) Fillings" you'll learn about the history of mercury amalgam (silver) fillings, including how they came to be and why the truth about them has taken so long to emerge. And you'll get an answer to a question I know you've thought about, which I've been asked a thousand times: "If the mercury released from these fillings is so toxic, why on earth are dentists still putting them in people's teeth?" What you'll learn will amaze you.

Two

A Brief History of Mercury Amalgam (Silver) Fillings

There's absolutely no doubt about it, *mercury vapor is released from amalgam fillings and is highly toxic to humans.* Yet nearly 50 percent of all general dentists still use them to fill cavities. But if amalgam fillings are so toxic, why did the dental profession decide to use them in the first place, and why on earth are dentists still putting them in people's teeth?

To answer these important questions, we need to journey back in time to discover how amalgam silver fillings came to be and explore the origins of the controversy. Turning the clock back will also help explain the role the American Dental Association (ADA) has played—and is still playing—in supporting the use of amalgams and controlling access to information about the health hazards these fillings pose.

Background

When amalgam fillings were first introduced in 1816, physicians and scientists questioned their safety. Even then, the medical and scientific community recognized mercury as a formidable poison and was aware that amalgam fillings contained mercury.

The problem was that, at the time, no one knew that amalgam fillings actually *released* poisonous mercury vapor. This is understandable because mercury vapor is an invisible, odorless gas. So even though the early proponents of amalgams readily acknowledged that mercury was a poison, no one could prove, or disprove, that the fillings released mercury. In fact, because the mixture of amalgam and silver resulted in a relatively hard substance, the pro-amalgam faction successfully argued that mercury was attached so tightly to the silver that it couldn't possibly escape the filling. Today—as yesterday—ignorance still fuels untruths!

But I'm getting ahead of myself . . . let's take a journey back in time to see where this all began.

The First Amalgam Filling

A Frenchman named Auguste Taveau created the first amalgam filling in 1816 when he mixed elemental mercury (the shiny, silvery liquid found in older thermometers) with shavings from silver coins. Then in 1830 two French brothers, the Crawcours, brought this silver filling material to England. The amalgam filling made the jump to America when the Crawcours emigrated to the U.S. in 1833. (The term "dentist" comes from the French word for tooth, *dent*. Interestingly, the amalgam filling was also invented in France.)

The term "amalgam" is not specific to dentistry. It actually describes a process by which elemental mercury is mixed with other metals to form a unique compound. In this case the mixture of the silver and mercury was called an amalgam. Essentially, the filling took the name of the process used to make it.

Those first amalgams were a great success. They contained approximately 50 percent elemental mercury and 50 percent silver filings. When mercury is mixed with silver it quickly forms a soft paste that can be easily packed into the hole (or cavity) in a tooth. The resultant paste remained pliable long enough to be inserted in the cavity and carved to fit the contours of the tooth before it hardened.

Prior to the invention of the amalgam filling, the most commonly used dental filling materials were thin sheets of lead that could be layered into a tooth's cavity and pounded together to fill the tooth. Other, less effective materials included cork, tin, wood chips, and various resins, such as pine.

Amalgam became the filling of choice simply because it was better than anything else available at the time—except for gold. However, gold was expensive and still hadn't been perfected as a filling material. So amalgam easily won out. It was inexpensive to produce, easy to mix and place, lasted longer, and sealed the tooth better than the alternatives. So it's easy to see why amalgam fillings became so popular.

But from the beginning this filling material was misnamed. A compound is normally named after its main ingredient. In the case of today's amalgams, the main ingredient is mercury, and silver is about 35 percent of the filling. Yet, for unknown reasons, this amalgamation of mercury and silver is still known as a silver or amalgam dental filling—*not* a *mercury* filling. The misnomer has no doubt contributed enormously to the continued popularity of amalgams. Certainly, far more people would be concerned about amalgam fillings if they knew the major ingredient was mercury. Even more would be concerned if they understood how toxic mercury is and how readily its vapor is released from amalgam fillings.

The Rest of the Story: The Controversy Begins

Prior to 1840, dentists fell into two categories: doctor-dentists, or physicians who also practiced dentistry, and barber-dentists. The term "barber-dentist" actually referred to a collection of tradesmen such as blacksmiths, silversmiths, cabinetmakers, and of course, barbers. Many of them moonlighted as pseudo-dentists who, until the invention of amalgams, were best known for cutting hair and pulling teeth. Old drawings depicting barber-dentists often showed a patient sitting in a barber's chair having a tooth pulled out—and not looking very happy about it.

The term "barber-dentists" likely became the popular name for this group because barbers had chairs for their clients (or should I say "victims") to sit in. As a result, they probably captured more of the dental market because early barber chairs had some adjustability, making it easier to work on the person's teeth. (James Snell invented the first reclining dental chair in 1832. But because barbers came before dentists, I've long suspected that the dental office chair was modeled after the barber chair.)

Mixing and placing amalgam fillings was so easy that barber-dentists took to it like ducks to water. When amalgams were first introduced, dental schools didn't exist. Literally anybody who could mix mercury and silver together could put these fillings into people's teeth and call themselves a barber-dentist, making a nice profit in the process. But not only were barber-dentists unregulated and untrained, no consumer protection laws existed to defend the patient from abuses, such as exposure to toxic substances and lack of sterilization. It was a chaotic situation at best.

Mad Hatter's Disease and Mercury

While barber-dentists couldn't care less about the mercury content of amalgam fillings, doctor-dentists (or physician-dentists, as they were also called) certainly did. Even in those days, the medical and scientific community knew that mercury was a poison. Proof was provided by observing the classic symptoms of chronic mercury poisoning exhibited by those who used elemental mercury in their profession—the hat makers.

In the 1800s nearly everyone wore hats, and "hatters" used a solution containing elemental mercury to turn fur into felt, the most common hat-making material of the time. But unbeknownst to the hatters, they were being continuously exposed to mercury vapor emitted from the felt-making solution. (Elemental mercury is the same form of mercury as used in amalgam fillings.)

If they worked at their trade long enough, all hatters eventually came down with a number of neurological symptoms that we now know are directly related to chronic mercury poisoning. This group's behavior was so bizarre that their condition was given a special name—Mad Hatter's disease. In reality, the hatters suffered from what I call "occupational mercury exposure" because it was their continuous/chronic exposure to mercury vapor that caused the symptoms related to this disease. The following lists some of the mercury-related neurological symptoms hatters experienced:

- tremors
- anxiety
- emotional instability
- mood swings
- irritability
- forgetfulness
- insomnia
- regressive behavior
- aggressiveness
- anger

Taken together, these symptoms made the hatters act in a strange and often crazy manner, thus the "mad" part of the disease name. The longer hatters were exposed to mercury vapor, the "madder" they became. Scientists eventually discovered that Mad Hatter's disease was directly related to chronic mercury poisoning, and I can imagine the physician-dentists were appalled when they learned that the elemental mercury used by hatters was the same type used in amalgam fillings.

But the medical community still had a problem they couldn't resolve. While physician-dentists knew that excessive exposure to elemental mercury could cause these symptoms, they didn't know mercury vapor could be released from a hardened amalgam. Nor did they yet understand how mercury did its damage. But the lack of specifics didn't stop doctors of that period from concluding that, because elemental mercury is a health hazard, amalgam fillings should be banned. Logical—and today we know how right they were.

Physician-Dentists Take Action

The doctor-dentists reasoned that if mercury could make hatters mad, it could do the same to those who had it in their teeth, being so close to the brain. Thus, doctor-dentists made it a priority to prevent barber-dentists from indiscriminately exposing the public to this poison.

But they discovered that stopping barber-dentists was easier said than done because it involved changing the heretofore unregulated practice of barber dentistry. The first obstacle was that they simply didn't have the power to make barber-dentists stop using amalgams. They overcame that dilemma by establishing the first dental school in the U.S in 1828—St. Francis Academy in Baltimore, Maryland, which in 1839 became the Baltimore College of Dental Surgery. In 1840 the first dental association, the American Society of Dental Surgeons (ASDS) was founded. Its purpose was to regulate and standardize dental treatment, give licensed dentists credibility and, more importantly, *prohibit the use of amalgam fillings by member dentists.*

Initially the ASDS flourished. It moved forward with its efforts against amalgam fillings and, in 1843, passed a resolution banning their use by any ASDS member. This well-intended resolution stated that members who continued to place amalgam fillings could lose their license to practice dentistry. While the resolution was wonderfully sensible, it had no effect on barber-dentists. Patients were still coming to them for amalgam fillings, they were making a lot of money, and they weren't at all concerned about the health hazards of mercury. So why worry about what the ASDS had to say? They didn't.

Where It All Went Wrong

It didn't take long for ASDS member dentists to realize they were losing patients to barber-dentists who were still offering the cheaper and longer-lasting amalgam fillings. Watching this sizable source of income slipping away, a significant number of ASDS dentists decided they wanted to use amalgam fillings and left the ASDS. As more and more dentists left the society, the ASDS saw the writing on the wall and disbanded for lack of members. It wasn't long after that the dentists who supported the use of amalgams got together to form their own dental association—the American Dental Association (ADA), founded in 1859. In effect, the ADA was formed so member dentists could generate revenues from placing amalgam fillings without fear of losing their licenses. This same association still regulates and controls the dental profession today—and continues to adamantly support the use of amalgams.

It's worth taking a few minutes to ponder the irony of this historic event. Under the ASDS, if a member dentist placed an amalgam filling, he could lose his license to practice dentistry. Acting from the known science and its concern for patient health, the ASDS did everything it could to protect the public from exposure to mercury. Today, under the ADA, if a dentist removes amalgam fillings because he or she supposedly "convinced" patients that the mercury released from their amalgams was a health hazard, the dentist could be censured, or even lose his or her license to practice dentistry. (I discuss the ADA's role and influence in detail in Chapter 13: "American Dental Association: Assessing the Blame.")

It's mind-boggling that in 1843 the medical profession was enlightened enough to recognize that mercury was poisonous (even though they couldn't prove it was released from amalgam fillings), and yet more than 150 years later, the ADA and its supporting pro-amalgam dentists remain in denial—even though it has been scientifically proven that amalgam fillings release mercury vapor.

Now is the time to revisit one of the questions that opened this chapter: "If amalgam fillings are so toxic, why did the dental profession decide to use them in the first place?" According to the ADA, the primary reasons were that they were easy to use and inexpensive. Certainly ignorance played a role, because the technology necessary to prove that mercury vapor is released from amalgams didn't exist at that time. But the course of events clearly shows that the profit motive ultimately led to the creation of the ADA and, from it, the continued use of these fillings today.

Fast Forward to the Present

Placed in a historical context, it's much easier to understand why little has changed regarding amalgam fillings from then until now. Today the ADA uses the following statements to defend its support of amalgam fillings:

- They have been used for over 150 years.
- They are durable.

- There is nothing that's better or more cost-effective.

- Hundreds of millions of people have them in their teeth.

While the ADA has always acknowledged that mercury is a poison, it has historically considered its presence in amalgam fillings a non-issue. This was because it believed that mercury was so chemically bound up with the other components of the filling that its toxic vapor couldn't possibly be released.

In fact, until recently the ADA has used that argument to defend its support for amalgam fillings. In 1984, due to overwhelming scientific evidence, the ADA finally admitted that mercury vapor is indeed released from amalgams. This should have ended the controversy, but as you'll learn, the ADA instead took a new position—one that simply cannot be defended (see Chapter 13).

Further Evidence

Since the time of amalgam's first introduction, many scientists, health professionals, anti-amalgam groups, patients, and an increasingly vocal group of mercury safe dentists have questioned the safety of these fillings. These concerned individuals and groups have aggressively challenged the ADA's contention that mercury fillings are not a health hazard. But even before it was scientifically proven that amalgams release mercury vapor, there were, and still are, other ways to demonstrate that they are hazardous to one's health.

An extensive amount of anecdotal, or subjective, evidence has proven that people with symptoms related to chronic mercury poisoning got better over time, *after* they had their amalgam fillings removed. However, the ADA doesn't consider anecdotal evidence to be scientific, and discounts it as not having any value or relevance.

I beg to differ. I've spoken to hundreds of patients who told me their health improved after having their amalgam fillings removed. It didn't matter to them whether the ADA found their improvement to be "unscientific." Chapter 12: "Health Improvements Related to Amalgam Removal and Mercury Detoxification" presents a number of significant studies showing health improvements after amalgam removal.

Thankfully, we no longer have to rely on anecdotal evidence to prove that amalgam fillings are a health hazard because it has been conclusively proven that mercury vapor *is* released from them. Confronted with that information, one would think the ADA would move quickly to ban these poisonous fillings. After all, why would it knowingly allow member dentists to continue to put mercury fillings into their patients' teeth when it has the power to immediately ban their use?

The ADA: Wrong Then—Wrong Now

But instead of banning their use, the ADA took an even more bizarre position. It claimed that the amount of vapor released wasn't enough to pose a health hazard to *anyone*, except the very small number of people who are allergic to mercury. According to the ADA's calculations, fewer than 100 people in the entire *world* are allergic to mercury. That erroneous and misleading assertion will be addressed later in the book.

The ADA was wrong 150 years ago when it said amalgam fillings didn't release mercury. And it is just as wrong today when it says that the mercury released from amalgams isn't a health hazard. What's even more amazing is that some pro-amalgam dentists, in spite of the ADA's admission to the contrary, continue to believe and tell patients that amalgams don't release mercury.

The Answer to the Second Question

It's time to answer the second question: If the mercury released from these fillings is so toxic, why on earth are dentists still putting them in people's teeth? I realize you've waited patiently for this answer and I'm sorry to disappoint you, but as hard as I've tried, I can't find a logical answer. But I can speculate.

Maybe the ADA is trying to save face. Maybe it's afraid of legal repercussions. Or maybe it truly believes mercury fillings are safe. Regardless of its reason, the ADA's stance still defies both logic and science. The fact is that there's no logical or scientific reason to continue using mercury fillings. Thousands of responsible scientists, and mercury free and mercury safe dentists, believe amalgam fillings are a health hazard because they release mercury vapor. Although placing amalgam fillings isn't currently illegal in many countries, in my opinion it's morally wrong. Safer and better filling materials are now available and, in comparison, amalgams can no longer be considered a good dental filling.

Yet, in spite of all of the scientific and anecdotal evidence to the contrary, the ADA and its pro-amalgam supporters continue to support the use, and safety, of mercury fillings. With its powerful lobby behind it, the ADA has so far been able to convince Congress and governmental regulatory agencies not to regulate the use of amalgams. But the tide is turning. As of the writing of this book, the anti-amalgam faction has made substantial inroads toward educating the public and encouraging Congress and the Federal Drug Administration (FDA) to stand up to the ADA and forever ban this poisonous dental material. I'm confident that as more and more information about these poisonous fillings becomes available to the public, the response to the ADA and its pro-amalgam supporters will be loud and clear—ban mercury amalgam fillings now!

Something to Think About

When I first began to explore this issue, the ADA's position shocked me. But I really wasn't surprised at the ignorance it has shown regarding the safety of amalgams. After all, history shows that scientists and health practitioners can get it very wrong. Take, for example, those who believed the sun revolved around the earth, and the earth was flat. Or the stance the medical profession took 500 years ago when it said that the blood didn't circulate in the body. And how about those who insisted that cigarette smoking didn't cause or contribute to lung cancer? These misguided claims were eventually overturned. The tragedy is that the health of hundreds of millions of people has been, and continues to be, harmed by the mercury released from these toxic fillings.

What's Next?

Knowing the history of mercury amalgam fillings and the role the ADA has played in supporting their use raises another question: Who is telling the truth? The ADA, or the ever-increasing number of mercury safe dentists who disagree with the ADA's position? To answer those questions we need to understand how amalgam fillings are made, how mercury vapor escapes from them, why they are a health hazard, and why they can *never* be considered safe or harmless.

Three

Mercury Amalgam (Silver) Fillings: What You Need to Know

One atom of mercury is poisonous to your body. That's right, just *one atom*! (An atom is the smallest part of an element that still retains its unique characteristics.) We're not talking about a truckload of mercury here. We're talking about a single, minute *atom* of mercury doing some harm to your body. The fact is that:

- Mercury is the most poisonous, naturally occurring, non-radioactive substance on the planet!

- *There is no safe level of mercury!*

- Amalgam fillings contain and release mercury as a poisonous vapor!

Eighty percent of the mercury vapor released from amalgam fillings is inhaled. Once inhaled, it passes quickly through the lungs, into and then out of the bloodstream, and accumulates in every cell of the body. As it accumulates, it poisons cells and tissues, particularly the brain and nervous system. This chapter will introduce you to mercury—the poison—not mercury the planet, or the astrological sign, or the car. By this chapter's end you'll understand why mercury is so poisonous and why amalgam fillings are extraordinarily hazardous to your health.

Three Types of Mercury

For all of this to make sense, a basic understanding of mercury is necessary. First of all, mercury is classified as a toxic metal—often called a "heavy metal."

The term "heavy" is added to "metal" because it refers to any metallic element that has a high density, or weight, and is poisonous in low concentrations. Mercury, being an element, cannot be broken down into anything else but mercury—and it cannot be destroyed or changed. Arsenic, lead, cadmium, nickel, and chromium are the most familiar of the toxic heavy metals. Everyone knows that arsenic is a deadly poison, and I doubt that anyone would consent to being exposed to it on a daily basis. Yet mercury is much more toxic than arsenic, and amalgam fillings release toxic doses of mercury throughout the day!

There are three types of mercury: organic, elemental, and inorganic.

- **Organic mercury** is mercury that is bonded to carbon in a methyl group (CH_3). This methyl, or hydrocarbon, unit is the basis of most organic compounds. Examples of organic mercury are methylmercury (CH_3Hg^+) and ethylmercury ($C_2H_5Hg^+$). Ethylmercury is the organic mercury compound found in the vaccine preservative thimerosal, which is believed by many to be the primary cause of, or contributor to, autism and other learning and developmental disorders. Organic mercury is also the type of mercury found in fish.

- **Elemental** or liquid mercury (Hg) refers to mercury in its pure, natural state—when it isn't combined with any other substance. In nature it rarely exists in its pure, elemental state and is found most often as cinnabar, a compound of mercury and sulfur (HgS). Cinnabar is mined and the pure mercury removed. Elemental mercury is the type used in amalgam fillings.

- **Inorganic** mercury is elemental mercury that is chemically bonded with other elements (excluding carbon) to form various compounds. An example is mercuric chloride ($HgCl_2$). This compound is, or has been, used in red tattoo dye, photography, skin bleaching creams, paints, preserving biological specimens, and treating syphilis.

While all forms of mercury are highly toxic, organic mercury is considered the most toxic, closely followed by elemental and then by inorganic mercury.

Unique Characteristics of Elemental Mercury

Elemental mercury is classified as a metal—but a metal with unique characteristics that sets it apart from all other metals. For example, mercury is the only metal that exists as a liquid at room temperature. And it's the only metal that gives off a colorless, tasteless, odorless, and deadly vapor at room temperature.

The vapor elemental mercury releases is one of the major reasons why it's so much more poisonous than any of the other heavy metals, such as lead and arsenic. For example, you can place a piece of lead on a table at room temperature, and it won't release lead vapor. Place room temperature mercury on a table, however, and it releases extremely high amounts of mercury vapor, 80 percent of which is absorbed into the lungs. Oddly enough, if you *swallow* elemental mercury, its toxicity is dramatically reduced. In its elemental form, only 0.01 percent of it is absorbed into the body from the intestine. The percentage of elemental mercury absorbed through the skin is also low—just 2 percent of what the lungs take in will penetrate the skin.

Another distinctive characteristic of mercury is that all the other metals except lead will dissolve in it. And this is the key to understanding the role mercury plays in the making of an amalgam filling. The amalgamation (mixing) of elemental mercury with powdered metals can be compared to the role water plays in making bread dough. The ingredients used in bread won't attach to each other without a solution that will hold everything together. Water is that catalyst for bread. When it's added to the other ingredients and mixed, everything binds together to form dough.

Mercury serves the same purpose with powdered metals. It acts as the catalyst, dissolving and binding the metals together to form the paste that can then be placed into a prepared cavity. Since amalgam's invention 1816, additional metals have been added to elemental mercury and silver filings, the original amalgam partners. These metals, in finely powdered form, were added to increase the filling's strength, reduce corrosion, and control expansion as it hardens. Today, an amalgam filling consists of approximately:

- elemental mercury (50%)
- powdered metals (50%)

The powdered metals are made up of approximately:

- 69% silver
- 26% tin
- 4% copper
- 1% zinc

The ratio of powdered metals will vary from manufacturer to manufacturer, but regardless of that ratio, **50 percent of the filling will still be elemental mercury**.

Remember . . . when you hear amalgam, *think mercury!* When you hear mercury, *think poison!*

So far so good, but we still need to address the question that stumped physician-dentists in the mid-1800s. How is it possible for an amalgam filling to release mercury?

How Mercury Vapor Escapes from Amalgam Fillings

For nearly 150, years pro-amalgam dentists believed that when mercury was mixed with other powdered metals and hardened, it couldn't release mercury. But even though an amalgam filling seems hard, mercury can escape from it because the chemical bond formed by mercury with silver, tin, zinc, and copper is actually very weak and unstable. In lay language, this means that when the amalgam is heated, the weak bond is readily broken. This allows elemental mercury to escape and pool on the surface of the filling, where it can then release its poisonous vapor.

At room temperature (68° F/20° C) the weak bond elemental mercury forms with the other metals will prevent it from escaping and releasing its vapor. But as the temperature of the filling increases, the bond is weakened further, increasing the amount of elemental mercury that escapes. For example, the temperature of the oral cavity is 98.6° F/37° C, and at this temperature mercury vapor will be released from the filling. *When it comes to amalgam fillings, think heat in . . . mercury vapor out!*

Temperature is the key to understanding how, and how much, mercury vapor an amalgam releases. Simply put, the amount of mercury released will be directly proportional to the temperature of the filling, along with how long it stays heated. Some protection against mercury vapor release from an unstimulated (at rest) amalgam filling is provided by the powdered metallic elements in the filling, such as tin and zinc, that combine with oxygen to form an oxide layer on the surface of an amalgam. This layer protects the filling from corrosion, but because it's very thin, it's easily removed by even the slightest abrasion, such as brushing, chewing gum, or eating.

But the amalgam filling itself isn't the problem, it's the vapor that is released from it. In fact, if you swallowed a piece of amalgam it wouldn't be toxic, because the contents of the stomach and intestine are essentially a liquid environment, which acts as a barrier that mercury vapor can't penetrate. Although some elemental mercury can be released by the action of stomach acid on amalgam particles, elemental mercury isn't well assimilated (0.01 percent) and therefore isn't a major concern.

Stimulating an Amalgam Filling

The temperature of an amalgam filling can be increased by many common forms of stimulation/friction, including chewing, brushing, teeth grinding, and drinking hot liquids. But those are just the everyday causes. Other forms of stimulation that raise the temperature of an amalgam include when it's removed by the dental drill or polished after placement. In addition, the temperature will dramatically increase when it comes into contact with an ultrasonic instrument commonly used to clean teeth.

But just how much vapor is released from elemental mercury at room temperature? At 68° F/20° C, if a container of elemental mercury was left open long enough to saturate the room, the concentration of mercury vapor in the air would reach 13,200 mcg/Hg/m³ (micrograms of mercury per cubic meter of air). The time it would take to saturate the room would depend on the size of the room, the temperature, and the amount of elemental mercury exposed to the air—but it wouldn't take very long. When it reaches the saturation point, it means that every cubic meter of air in that room would contain 13,200 mcg of mercury. As you'll soon learn, that's an extraordinarily large number of mercury atoms! In fact, if the room was monitored by a regulatory agency, the alarms would be blaring long before this level was reached.

If you put your nose five to six inches away from the open container of mercury and inhaled for even a few minutes, you would quickly experience symptoms related to acute mercury exposure, very likely requiring emergency attention.

Understanding how mercury vapor is released from an amalgam filling is the key to understanding why these fillings are so toxic and so hazardous to your health. With that in mind, it's time to find out how much mercury is too much mercury—I guarantee it will be an eye opener.

How Much is Too Much?

Science has proven that just one atom of mercury is toxic. So how can anyone say that the amount of mercury an amalgam filling releases is too small to be harmful? The ADA and its pro-amalgam supporters say amalgams don't release enough mercury to be harmful, so it looks like we have a serious contradiction here. After all, if one atom of mercury is toxic to the body, then it's logical to assume that 100 or 1 million atoms would be even more so. In order to attach numbers to mercury atoms, we need to begin by defining a microgram (mcg), because mercury isn't just toxic in ounces, grams, or milligrams—but in *micrograms* (mcg).

To grasp the size of a microgram, it's helpful to relate it to something more familiar. As you'll see, a microgram is extremely small compared to an ounce—

or even to a gram or a milligram. But as small as a microgram is, it still contains astronomical amounts of mercury atoms.

On their own, the numbers 3 mcg, 20 mcg, or 50 mcg may not seem like much. But how do the numbers 12 trillion, 80 trillion, and 200 trillion sound to you? When you recall that every atom of mercury that accumulates in your body will harm it in some way, those numbers can ***never*** be considered too small not to worry about. *There are actually more atoms of mercury in just 30 micrograms than there are cells in the human body.* This number is astonishing when you realize that the body is made up of about 100 trillion cells (a trillion is a 1 with 12 zeros after it).

Number of Mercury Atoms in a Microgram	
Unit of Measure	*Contains*
One ounce	28 grams (gm)
One gram	1,000 milligrams (mg)
One milligram	1,000 micrograms (mcg)
Atoms of mercury in one microgram	4,000,000,000,000 (4 trillion)

Further Exploration

But let's explore this further. We inhale about 80 percent of the mercury vapor amalgam fillings release. For example, if you had an amalgam filling and it released 10 mcg of mercury vapor per cubic meter of air per hour (10 mcg/Hg/m^3/hr), your body would absorb about 8 mcg of mercury per hour. I'll do the math for you.

10 mcg/Hg/m^3/hr x 80% = 8 mcg/Hg/hr . . . or 32 trillion atoms!

If you wanted to know the amount that you'd take in after 30 minutes of breathing in that amount of mercury vapor, you'd divide the 8 by ½, which is 4 mcg of mercury per hour. Or if you wanted to know the amount of mercury absorbed in 24 hours, you'd simply multiply 8 by 24, which is 192 mcg of mercury. However many micrograms of mercury you take in, you will have to multiply each microgram by 4 trillion to get the total number of mercury atoms.

You don't have to be a mathematician to comprehend these numbers. It becomes even more significant when your realize that in the United States, the average person has 10 amalgam fillings. The estimated amount of mercury in 10 amalgam fillings is 5 grams, or 5 million micrograms. When you multiply that by 4 trillion, you'll see that it's a *lot* of mercury to be carrying around in your teeth!

From Very Small to Very Large

As you've seen, we started with something that at first glance appeared to be very, very small (10 mcg of mercury released from a filling) and watched it turn into an extraordinarily large amount—32 trillion. This means your body will have one heck of a lot of mercury atoms to deal with every minute of every day for as long as the fillings are in your teeth. The human body has an amazing capacity for punishment, and it has the miraculous ability—up to a point—to remove small amounts of mercury every day. But under this continuous onslaught of mercury, your body becomes less and less effective at removing it over time.

Of interest here is that an American Dental Association media release, from July 2002, stated the following: "Minute amounts of mercury vapor (between 1–3 micrograms per day) may be released from amalgam under the pressure of chewing or tooth grinding (also called Bruxism), but there is no scientific evidence that such low-level exposure is harmful."

Again, I beg to differ. Scientific studies have conclusively shown the amount released to be much higher than the ADA's estimates, but at least it agrees that mercury vapor is released from amalgams. I believe that if anyone, including the ADA, says these fillings are not a health hazard, they should take the time to do the math. If so, they would never again think that even 3 mcg of mercury per day would be too small to constitute a health hazard.

Factors Determining the Amount of Mercury Vapor Released

A number of factors must be considered when determining how much mercury vapor amalgam fillings release daily. (Please note that the conditions in the mouth vary greatly, and even two people of equal age and health, with identical fillings, can release different amounts of mercury vapor over the same period of time.) The following factors determine the amount of mercury a person would be exposed to:

- the type of amalgam; high or low copper content
- the number of fillings
- how long they've been in the teeth
- how and how often they are stimulated
- how long the stimulation lasts

For example, while a person is chewing gum, the amount of mercury vapor released is relatively high. After chewing ends, it takes about 90 minutes for the filling to cool down and the vapor levels to decrease to the unstimulated level. Many variations on this basic theme exist. For example, if a person chews gum for 30 minutes, he or she will be exposed to more mercury during those 30 minutes than another person with the same number of mercury fillings who chews gum for 15 minutes.

Along the same line, if someone snacks frequently, their exposure to mercury is greater than someone who doesn't snack, given the same number of fillings. And those who grind their teeth will be exposed to significantly more mercury than those who don't, even though they all have the same number of fillings. (High copper amalgams, introduced in the late 1960s, release 50 times more mercury in a given period of time than the older low-copper amalgams.)

Common Sources of Mercury Exposure

In 1991, the World Health Organization (WHO) estimated the amount of mercury taken in daily by the body from a variety of sources, along with the type of mercury. Here's what the WHO discovered.

WHO's Source of Mercury Exposure		
Source	Average Daily Exposure	Type
Amalgam fillings	3–17 mcg	Elemental mercury
Fish and seafood	2.3 mcg	Methyl mercury
Other food	0.3 mcg	Inorganic mercury
Air and water	Negligible traces	All types

People with amalgam fillings will receive more mercury from their fillings than from all the other sources of mercury combined. But while amalgam fillings top the WHO list, you can also see that it's not the only source of mercury. To accurately evaluate the harm mercury is doing to your health, you must consider all sources, particularly fish and occupational exposure, which can significantly add to the amount received from amalgam fillings. (Remember, the WHO statistics are averages, and tens of millions of people will be exposed to much higher daily amounts of mercury from their amalgam fillings.)

Proof that Mercury Vapor is Released

Another question I'm often asked is, "How can you *prove* that mercury is released from amalgam fillings?" This is a legitimate, insightful, and important question. Scientists have used a number of instruments and methods to verify that mercury vapor is released from amalgams, including mercury vapor gas analyzers, the electron-dispersive X-ray analysis, and a diffusive sampler. Sure, they sound pretty complicated and expensive—and they are. The least expensive and easiest to use is the Jerome mercury vapor analyzer. Regulatory agencies, businesses, and mercury safe dentists use this instrument to measure and monitor mercury vapor at facilities/dental offices where employees/patients could be exposed to mercury. It can also be used to measure the release of mercury vapor from amalgam fillings before, during, and after stimulation.

In my opinion, Arizona Instruments makes the best mercury vapor analyzer. I've used their Jerome Mercury Vapor Analyzer extensively to measure the amount of mercury vapor released from amalgam fillings during different methods of stimulation. I like it because it meets industry standards, is portable, and accurately measures mercury vapor levels in the air as small as 0.003 mcg/Hg/m³ and as high as 999 mcg/Hg/m³ (micrograms of mercury per cubic meter of air). Information about Arizona Instruments is found in Appendix D.

The Toothbrushing Test

I'll describe a test I've done numerous times, the results of which conclusively demonstrate that mercury vapor is released from these fillings. For testing purposes, I used an extracted tooth with a three-surface amalgam filling (top and two sides). A pre-stimulation sample of air was taken directly above the filling, to be used as a reference. The Jerome Mercury Vapor Analyzer detected no mercury vapor being released at room temperature.

The occlusal (top) surface of the filling was then brushed with a soft bristle toothbrush, with no toothpaste, for 10 seconds. The Jerome analyzer was then used to test the air directly above the filling for mercury vapor. Depending on how much pressure was applied to the filling by the bristles, the results varied, ranging from 350 mcg/Hg/m³ to a high of 500 mcg/Hg/m³. That's the amount of mercury vapor released from brushing just one amalgam filling for just 10 seconds! If this brushing test were performed in someone's mouth, the amount of mercury vapor released would vary depending on many factors, including:

- the type of brush (hard, medium, or soft)
- the brushing pressure
- how long the fillings were brushed
- the number of amalgam fillings that were brushed
- type of amalgam; high or low copper content

- the size of the fillings

- the amount of saliva present

The presence of saliva, for example, can result in a lower mercury vapor reading because saliva can capture some of the mercury vapor, making it unavailable to the analyzer for recording. But just because it isn't recorded doesn't mean you're home free. Mercury vapor captured by saliva can be converted to highly toxic organic mercury—in both the mouth and intestine by bacteria. This isn't good news, because the organic mercury that finds its way into the intestine will be nearly 100 percent assimilated into the body. So although the Jerome analyzer is highly accurate for mercury vapor, if it's used to record mercury vapor levels in the mouth, it won't record all of the mercury released during the testing period.

It is one thing to test for mercury vapor released when the filling is stimulated and another to monitor the dental office for mercury vapor. Because no regulatory agency has seen fit to monitor the dental office, I consider the Jerome Mercury Vapor Analyzer a must-have for every dental practice.

The Video

An amazing video produced by the International Academy of Oral Medicine and Toxicology (IAOMT) actually *shows* mercury vapor coming off an amalgam filling. Mercury vapor is invisible to the human eye but casts a shadow in black light, allowing it to be filmed. The IAOMT video offers undeniable visual proof that amalgams release mercury vapor. You can access it on my website, www. dentalwellness4u.com, under the FAQ menu on the homepage.

Galvanic Current

If both amalgam fillings and gold crowns are present in the mouth at the same time—a *very* common occurrence—a galvanic current (similar to what happens in a car battery) is generated between the two distinct metal fillings. This current causes the continuous release of mercury, even when the amalgam fillings are not being stimulated. In essence, even if your fillings were never heated you would still be exposed to mercury vapor from them 24 hours a day! Thus, the galvanic effect is very significant when determining your *total* exposure to mercury from amalgams.

One study showed that samples of gum tissue taken during oral surgery on patients with 6 or more amalgam fillings contained 20 times the mercury levels of patients in the control group. The researchers concluded that this was caused by galvanic action between gold restorations and amalgam fillings. Another significant study by Hanson and Pleva reported that from 30 to 60 micrograms of mercury can be released per day, due to galvanic current between a gold crown and an amalgam—from just one amalgam filling. As you now know, this is a significant amount of mercury.

Types of Stimulation and Mercury Vapor Released

A number of researchers have examined how much mercury vapor amalgam fillings release during various forms of stimulation. The following table shows the results of a study by Malmström et al.

Types of Stimulation and Mercury Vapor Released	
Condition or Stimulation	*Amount of Hg* Released*
Amalgam fillings at rest	36 mcg/Hg/m³**
Chewing food	68 mcg/Hg/m³
Eating sweets	70 mcg/Hg/m³
Toothbrushing	272 mcg/Hg/m³
Polishing amalgams after a dental cleaning***	504 mcg/Hg/m³
Wet (water cooled) polishing an amalgam filling***	597 mcg/Hg/m³
Dry polishing an amalgam filling***	4,295 mcg/Hg/m³

* Hg is the symbol for mercury   ** m³ is a cubic meter of air   *** Stimulation initiated at a dental office

As you see, significant amounts of mercury vapor can be released during some very common forms of amalgam stimulation. But what about during the removal process? Drilling out just one average sized amalgam filling can release up to 4,000 mcg/Hg/m³ of mercury vapor. This will help you understand why I promote the safe removal of amalgam fillings!

Malmström's study, and other pertinent tests, prove beyond the shadow of any doubt that mercury vapor is released from amalgam fillings—**and in significant amounts**. In addition, these tests also prove that different forms of filling stimulation will cause differing amounts of mercury vapor to be released.

A Comparison to Regulatory Guidelines for Mercury

You've learned a great deal about mercury and how much can be released by the many common forms of amalgam filling stimulation. Now it's time to put it into context by comparing these amounts to mercury exposure levels at the workplace. All agencies that monitor occupational safety levels for mercury universally agree that mercury vapor is highly toxic. Because the use of mercury in various industrial products creates a risk of mercury exposure to employees, a number of agencies have established guidelines to monitor and protect workers. For example, if the monitored air exceeds the "safe" level of mercury, employees must leave the area of exposure.

These attempts to set a "safe" level for mercury are an official acknowledgement that, regardless of the source, mercury vapor is a health hazard at even extremely low levels. But understand, these agencies aren't saying mercury is safe, only that a majority of the people won't show obvious signs of mercury poisoning while at the workplace if they are exposed to the arbitrary daily levels established. As you will see, monitoring agencies don't all agree on what the so-called "safe" level should be.

Regulatory Standards

The guidelines set by these agencies, except for the Agency for Toxic Substances and Disease Registry (ASTDR), only monitor occupational mercury exposure at the workplace and are based on a 40-hour work week. While these guidelines are great for monitoring mercury exposure during the workday, over 150 million people with amalgam fillings in the United States are being exposed to mercury 24 hours a day, 365 days a year. No regulatory agency has factored mercury vapor released from amalgams into the equation when monitoring employees' exposure to mercury. Each agency only monitors the air for mercury at the workplace, not the air inside an employee's oral cavity. None of the guidelines have been adjusted to take into account employees' exposure to mercury from contaminated fish, and environmental sources outside of the workplace.

National Institute for Occupational Safety and Health (NIOSH) www.cdc.gov/niosh

NIOSH sets its exposure limit at 50 mcg/Hg/m^3 of mercury per cubic meter of air as a time-weighted average (TWA) for up to a 10-hour workday and a 40-hour workweek. TWA means the levels are regularly tested and the average is used to determine mercury levels in the air.

Occupational Safety and Health Administration (OSHA) www.osha.gov

OSHA guidelines are the same exposure levels set by NIOSH.

World Health Organization (WHO) www.who.int/en

The WHO limit for occupational exposure to mercury vapor is 25 mcg/Hg/m^3 per 8-hour shift.

Agency for Toxic Substances and Disease Registry (ATSDR) www.atsdr.cdc.gov

The ATSDR set a minimal risk level (MRL) for chronic exposure to mercury vapor at 3 mcg/Hg/m³ per hour over a 24-hour period. The ATSDR concluded that 3 mcg/m³ per hour is the amount of mercury vapor a person can be continuously exposed over a 24-hour period without showing any observable side effects.

More information about these agencies can be found on their websites, or by going to www.dentalwellness4u.com and selecting the top row menu: Layperson Info. The ADA continues to lobby the regulatory agencies that mercury amalgams are safe and the mercury released from them doesn't pose a health hazard. It doesn't take a lot of imagination to understand why the ADA doesn't want the regulatory agencies monitoring the dental offices and the mouths of people with amalgam fillings.

The ADA's Position

It's time to take a closer look at the ADA's position on mercury fillings. The ADA claims that unless a patient is *allergic* to mercury, *no one with amalgam fillings will ever be exposed to harmful levels of mercury.* The ADA steadfastly insists that mercury fillings are not hazardous to your health, and that you don't have to be concerned about having them in your teeth or in the teeth of your children.

But how does the ADA's position compare to what you've learned so far? Let's review.

- Even one atom of mercury harms the body.
- An enormous number of toxic mercury atoms are contained in very small amounts of mercury.
- Mercury vapor is released from unstimulated amalgam fillings.
- Large amounts of mercury vapor are released when amalgam fillings are stimulated.
- The amount of mercury vapor released can vary dramatically, depending on factors such as number, size, how long the fillings are in the teeth, the type of the amalgam, and the duration of the stimulation.
- Mercury vapor is continuously released until the stimulation has ceased and the fillings have cooled down—up to 90 minutes.
- People who grind their teeth at night will continuously be exposed to high amounts of mercury vapor, as well as throughout the day via other forms of stimulation.

● Galvanic action between gold and amalgam fillings can cause a constant release of mercury, even when they haven't been stimulated.

What you've learned so far regarding mercury vapor and what the ADA claims about it are vastly different. The ADA says the amount of mercury released from fillings is harmless, but science says otherwise. And there's even more evidence, so let's take this one step further.

Teeth as Hazardous Waste Containers

In 1988, the Environmental Protection Agency (EPA) labeled the materials used in dental amalgams, and the amalgam particles removed from them, as toxic waste material. Under these regulations, when the two components of amalgam— elemental mercury and powdered metals—are delivered to the dental office, they must be placed in a hazardous waste container. Additionally, any excess amalgam left over after a filling is put in or replaced must also be put into a hazardous waste container. Any dental school or dental office that doesn't comply with the EPA's regulations regarding the handling of these materials is subject to a fine.

Think about it. *The EPA considers the materials that make up an amalgam filling—and the amalgam filling itself—toxic waste.* But now we come to the scary part. If the components of an amalgam filling, and the filling itself, are considered hazardous waste—what does that make the teeth they are put into? That's right. It makes them *hazardous waste containers*! Even worse, these waste containers don't have a lid, and you're forced to take them with you wherever you go.

OSHA Requirements

The Occupational Safety and Health Administration (OSHA) requires that dental office staff handle discarded amalgam in the following manner:

● The staff must use a "no touch" technique for handling amalgam, meaning no one should handle amalgam without protection.

● Amalgam must be stored away from heat in unbreakable, tightly sealed hazardous waste containers.

● Amalgam waste particles must be covered with liquid to eliminate the risk of exposing the office staff to mercury vapor.

These regulations make complete sense. But imagine if they were extended to the amalgams in your teeth. It would mean that you couldn't touch your fillings without first putting on gloves. You'd have to cover your tongue before it touched the fillings, and you'd be required to keep your teeth covered with a protective liquid 24/7!

Banning a Poison

Mercury is a powerful poison, and accordingly its use has been banned in many products. For example, in 1990 the EPA banned the use of mercury in latex house paints. Mercurochrome, a household item once commonly used for cuts and scrapes, was banned because it contained mercury. Thermometers and blood pressure kits containing elemental mercury are being phased out, or have already been banned, in many states and countries. Mercury has been banned from numerous products, but not from the human mouth.

At the time this book went to press, a number of cities throughout the U.S. and Canada—including San Francisco, Duluth, Seattle, Montreal, Victoria, and Toronto—had passed laws banning the sale, import, or manufacture of products containing mercury. A number of cities and counties regulate the discharge of amalgam waste particles from dental offices into the wastewater. This last fact points up another absurdity—mercury and amalgam particles can't be put into wastewater—but are allowed in your teeth.

Manufacturers of amalgam filling material are also getting the message. Degussa AG, at one time the largest amalgam producer in Germany, no longer makes amalgam filling material. Degussa didn't offer a reason for their decision, but a logical deduction would be that the company wanted to protect itself against possible legal action. In addition, Kerr and Dentsply/Caulk, two U.S. companies that manufacture dental amalgam, have issued a list of contraindications for the use of amalgam as a dental filling, including the well-known side effects of chronic mercury poisoning, in their amalgam packaging.

Everyone Except the Business of Dentistry

Every business that uses mercury is regulated and monitored by numerous regulatory agencies except one—*dental offices*. It seems that just about everyone is in agreement about regulating and monitoring mercury—except the ADA and pro-amalgam dentists. Facilities that use mercury are required to continuously monitor the amount of mercury vapor present using very accurate instruments. If the amount exceeds the regulatory standards, the business is closed down and employees evacuated, until the levels are considered "safe." That's what you'd expect from regulatory agencies created to protect you and the environment from toxic substances.

But for reasons that I've never been able to discover, dentistry is the only business/industry using mercury that isn't required to abide by these regulations. Yet when an amalgam is placed, drilled out, or polished, it releases enormous amounts of mercury vapor. In most pro-amalgam dental offices, amalgam fillings are being placed, removed, replaced, and polished on a daily basis. Unless protective measures are taken, the amount of mercury vapor released during these dental procedures will far exceed the maximum allowed in any workplace using mercury.

The EPA estimates that 1,088 tons of mercury—55 percent of the mercury in use today in the U.S.—is contained in dental fillings. In addition, 34 tons of mercury are added to this total *each year* from the placement of new amalgam fillings. The mercury used in dental offices that don't have amalgam separators to capture mercury in the wastewater ends up in the environment.

In addition, over 150 million people in the United States eliminate varying amounts of mercury daily via urine and feces. All of this goes into the wastewater and must be included in the total environmental load of mercury from amalgams. This makes dentists one of the largest users, and polluters, of mercury—and yet it's the *only business that isn't regulated and monitored!* I challenge anyone to explain the reasoning behind that!

Why aren't dental offices regulated and why aren't patients, dentists, office staff, and wastewater being monitored by a regulatory agency? It would seem the logical thing to do. But instead of protecting you from these toxic fillings, the ADA uses its vast lobbying network to influence regulatory agencies not to monitor or regulate dental offices or ban amalgam fillings.

The Danger of Omission

In order to make an educated decision about amalgam fillings, you need to know certain facts. And if your dentist is pro-amalgam, you've probably never been offered this information. These dentists omit key facts because they don't know them, they don't consider them important, or they believe the ADA's position on amalgams. But *every* dentist takes an oath to provide patients with information needed to protect their patients' oral and overall health. Thus, I believe all dentists are obligated to disclose the following information before placing an amalgam filling:

- An amalgam (silver) filling is 50 percent mercury.

- Mercury vapor is released from amalgam fillings and puts every aspect of your health at risk.

- Mercury vapor released from your amalgam fillings will expose the fetus and nursing baby to high amounts of mercury and endanger his or her health.

- Mercury is vastly more toxic to the fetus and developing child than to adults.

- Tens of millions of people are allergic or sensitive to mercury, and you should consider being tested for a mercury allergy.

- Common actions such as eating, gum chewing, tooth brushing, and tooth grinding can dramatically increase the release of mercury vapor from your amalgam fillings.

- Diet, the environment, or your occupational exposure to mercury could significantly add to the amount you're already receiving from amalgam fillings.

- If you're in poor health, even minute amounts of mercury could have a damaging effect on your immune system and decrease your body's ability to resist free radicals and toxins.

- The mercury vapor released from your amalgam fillings accumulates in your body.

- The EPA considers the components and pieces of an amalgam filling toxic waste.

Every dentist should then do the following:

- Recommend that you be tested for mercury poisoning.

- Suggest a mercury detoxification program to remove mercury from your body.

- Ask you to sign a release form giving your consent for him or her to expose you, or your children, to mercury.

If your dentist had properly disclosed all of this information, I doubt you would have ever consented to having mercury fillings put into your teeth.

Mercury Risk Evaluation

Given what you've read so far, you may be wondering just what your risk of chronic mercury poisoning is. Over the years, many people have asked me how they could evaluate the *extent* of their mercury exposure. In response, I've created a simple risk evaluation to help determine a person's exposure to mercury. It consists of three risk categories—low, moderate, and high—and is based on your own subjective self-evaluation. The evaluation not only considers your exposure to mercury from your amalgam fillings, but also other sources of mercury exposure, as well as your present health status.

I recommend that you take this evaluation even if you haven't yet experienced any mercury-related symptoms. It will give you a good idea as to where you are now—and the direction you're heading. You can take the evaluation by going to my website, www.dentalwellness4u.com, and clicking on "Mercury Risk Evaluation" in the Frequently Asked Questions (FAQ) menu. While this isn't an objective evaluation, I'm sure you'll find it interesting. (Appendix A discusses the objective tests for mercury.)

A Quick Review

It doesn't matter where your exposure to mercury originates—be it amalgam fillings, contaminated fish, environmental pollution, or a broken thermometer—it's still mercury. All forms of mercury are poisonous and can't be called *harmful* when the source is contaminated fish or occupational exposure, and then deemed *harmless* when it is emitted from amalgam fillings.

There is no such thing as "good mercury." *Mercury is a poison regardless of its source.* The body has no biological need for it. Once you fully grasp the fact that there is *no such thing as a safe or harmless level of mercury*, the door to understanding why amalgam fillings are so hazardous to your health will full open.

What's Next?

It's one thing to understand that mercury is a powerful poison and that amalgam fillings release large amounts of it. It's another thing altogether to understand that the mercury that enters your body and accumulates there can have a serious impact on your health over time. The next chapter will put it all together for you.

Four

Chronic Mercury Poisoning and Amalgam (Silver) Fillings

Everyone who has amalgam fillings is being poisoned by mercury. The mercury that's emitted as a vapor from them doesn't just vanish into the air—80 percent of it enters your body, accumulates over time, and will negatively affect your health. That said, let's take a look at why mercury is so poisonous and the role amalgam fillings play in chronic mercury poisoning.

Acute and Chronic Mercury Poisoning

Mercury poisoning is always classified as either "acute" or "chronic," but there are degrees of both. The damage mercury can do to your health, acutely or chronically, is directly related to the following:

- the type of mercury
- the amount of exposure
- the length of exposure
- how much has accumulated in the body
- where it's stored in the body

- when you were first exposed to it

- how long it's been there

- the health of your immune/detoxification system

Acute Mercury Poisoning

Acute mercury poisoning is relatively rare and occurs when you've been exposed to a sudden and very high dose of mercury, mainly from elemental mercury vapor or organic mercury. This type of exposure will cause rapid and severe symptoms, requiring immediate attention. Some of the more intense symptoms that will occur soon after exposure include:

- tightness in the chest

- severe chest pains

- nausea

- acute tiredness and malaise

- severe cough

- excessive salivation

- diarrhea

- shortness of breath

- tremors

- chills

- severe abdominal pains

- headaches

If an acute dose of mercury is high enough and left untreated, it can lead to death in a short period of time due to kidney (renal) failure, heart attack, or pneumonia. Acute mercury poisoning is the kind that physicians and emergency rooms are most familiar with, and are trained to treat.

Chronic Mercury Poisoning

In contrast, chronic mercury poisoning is very common, still largely unrecognized, and definitely under-diagnosed. It's caused by continuous exposure to low levels of mercury over an extended period of time, such as the exposure to mercury vapor from amalgam fillings. If mercury enters the body and accumulates faster than the body can remove it, it will gradually build up until the body becomes mercury toxic. At that point the individual will experience an observable symptom. Unless the source of mercury is removed, more and more symptoms related to chronic mercury poisoning will appear over time.

Since so many factors determine the extent of a person's exposure to mercury, the time it takes for early symptoms of chronic mercury poisoning to appear will vary greatly. Depending on the degree and length of one's exposure to mercury, it could take years before enough of it has accumulated to manifest a noticeable symptom.

Initially, early symptoms of chronic mercury poisoning may come and go. Because many mercury-related symptoms are so common, it's unlikely that you or your doctor will initially associate them with mercury toxicity. For example, did you ever consider that headaches, memory loss, fatigue, digestive disorders, ringing in the ears, and depression—to name but a few symptoms—are related to mercury poisoning?

While the onset of chronic mercury poisoning isn't as sudden or intense as acute mercury poisoning, over time it can be very destructive to your overall health, and can eventually contribute to many life-threatening illnesses. In fact, most dentists and health professionals aren't aware of the wide range of symptoms that are directly and indirectly related to chronic mercury poisoning. You'll find a list of the most common symptoms and diseases in Chapter 5: "Symptoms and Diseases Related to Chronic Mercury Poisoning."

While it's not apples to apples, comparing mercury poisoning to radiation poisoning will help you understand how the chronic form differs from the acute form. Take a lethal radiation leak. Those in the immediate area of the leak would likely receive an acute and fatal dose. But those individuals far enough away from the main source wouldn't receive a fatal dose. Depending on how long they were exposed to a lower dose, and the total dose received, they could manifest a radiation-related illness related to a chronic exposure at a later date. Over time, serious health problems could appear, possibly contributing to premature death.

The same principles apply to the relationship between acute and chronic mercury poisoning. If you're exposed to a sudden and very high dose of organic or elemental mercury and aren't treated quickly, you could die. If you are continuously exposed to small doses of mercury, it won't kill you immediately, but you'll ultimately manifest symptoms of mercury poisoning and, over time, it can seriously damage your health and shorten your life expectancy.

The Many Faces of Chronic Mercury Poisoning

As mercury continues to accumulate in the body it can contribute to, or make worse, every known health problem. Mercury negatively impacts your health because it can:

- Attach to essential proteins, enzymes, and other vital substances and interfere with their normal function.

- Make you more susceptible to autoimmune diseases and allergies.

- Cause allergic reactions (mercury is an allergen).

- Interfere with the body's ability to make hemoglobin and hemoglobin's ability to carry oxygen.

- Damage the cardiovascular system.

- Interfere with the natural detoxification pathways of the liver, kidneys, skin, and intestine.

- Cause intestinal bacteria and yeast, including Candida, to become immune to mercury, making them resistant to antibiotic and antifungal treatment.

- Deplete the body of its most important antioxidants and severely weaken all aspects of the immune system.

Where the Mercury Goes

The body is comprised of trillions of cells—and mercury can easily enter *every one of them.* This characteristic also explains why so many symptoms are associated with chronic mercury poisoning. According to estimates, there are at least 100 related symptoms.

Mercury can interfere with every body system, both directly and indirectly, and this is more example of why it's such a potent a poison.

Systems of the Body Affected by Mercury	
Immune	Reproductive
Nervous	Urinary
Endocrine	Digestive
Circulatory	Lymphatic
Muscular	Skeletal

Mercury's broad distribution throughout the body also speaks to why the appearance of symptoms related to chronic mercury poisoning could be delayed for years. In effect, mercury is so widely dispersed that it can take a long period of time for enough to accumulate in any one location, or system, for a recognizable symptom to manifest. Of course, the bad news is that the cells and tissues of your body are still being poisoned every single day.

However, if mercury had an affinity for only one organ, the effect would be much more severe and would appear much sooner. For example, if all the mercury entering the body daily from amalgam fillings only went to the thyroid gland, you would quickly see an observable symptom related to thyroid function.

What Makes Mercury So Poisonous?

First, mercury can easily enter every cell of the body. Second, it damages proteins and enzymes. Third, it generates enormous amounts of toxic free radicals. But let's first look at *why* mercury is so adept at sneaking into cells.

The membranes that surround all cells (and those that surround numerous compartments within the cells) are composed mainly of fatty substances, interspersed with proteins. This fatty membrane is an important protective mechanism against unwanted substances. The fatty wall of the cell acts like a barrier, with many security gates. Anything that wants to enter the cell must be escorted through these gates by the various proteins that transport substances in and out of the cell.

But as it turns out, elemental mercury vapor is highly fat soluble. This characteristic allows it to readily pass through the membrane of every cell in the body, easily bypassing the guardians of the cell membrane. Additionally, mercury has no problem crossing the critical blood-brain barrier (the lining of protective blood capillaries surrounding the brain). Mercury can pass into the brain by penetrating the tightly packed, highly specialized, fat-lined endothelia cells that make up the lining.

It isn't just mercury's ability to effortlessly pass through the cell membrane that makes it so destructive. It's the fact that it now has direct access to the cellular components that are so vital to cellular health and function. Mercury alters the function of cellular proteins and enzymes, along with any cellular component that contains protein as part of its structure. A quick primer on amino acids, proteins, and enzymes will help you understand how this works.

Amino Acids, Proteins, and Enzymes

Amino acids

Amino acids are a unique class of nitrogen-containing acids. There are 10 nonessential and 10 essential amino acids. Nonessential amino acids can be made by the body from other amino acids. Essential amino acids can't be manufactured by the body and must be obtained from food sources or supplements. But *all* amino acids are considered necessary to sustain life. (Don't be confused by the term "nonessential." This is the term scientists use to describe the amino acids that the body can manufacture on its own, but these 10 are still absolutely essential.)

Various combinations of the 20 amino acids are strung together in unique sequences to form protein and peptide chains. Chains of over 50 amino acids are referred to as "proteins," such as hemoglobin, collagen, and myosin (a muscle protein). Chains of less than 50 amino acids are called "peptides," actually very small proteins, such as insulin and the antioxidant glutathione. Glutathione is also known by its acronym, GSH. Every protein manufactured by the body and all of the 20 amino acids are necessary for good health.

Cysteine and Methionine

While proteins contain numerous combinations of many amino acids, most will also contain significant numbers of two very important amino acids—*cysteine* and *methionine*. Depending on the size of the protein, it could contain hundreds of these two amino acids. What makes these two special is that they are the only amino acids of the 20 that have a distinct sulfur component. And mercury has a very powerful attraction to the sulfur part of these amino acids. Cysteine is also a key component of the body's most important and prevalent mercury chelator, glutathione (GSH). (The sulfur part of an amino acid is called a thiol, or sulfhydryl group.)

A chelator (chelating agent) is a substance that binds with various materials, both harmful and essential, and facilitates their removal from the body. Chelators, such as glutathione, are produced by the body, found naturally in foods and supplements, or can be pharmaceutical agents, e.g., DMSA (Dimercaptosuccinic Acid) and DMPS (2,3-Dimercapto-1-propanesulfonic acid).

Proteins

Proteins are the key to the structure, function, regulation, and health of *all* cells. According to estimates, a single cell can contain up to one billion protein molecules, each of which can contain from 50 to 5,000 amino acids. Proteins are indispensable for transporting essential materials between cells and for communicating within and between them, especially in the brain. Most of the critical components found in the cell and necessary for cellular health are made of proteins, such as enzymes, antioxidants, antibodies, hormones, and DNA.

Mercury damages proteins because it displaces the essential minerals that normally attach to the sulfhydryl group, such as zinc, copper, magnesium, iron, and iodine, and then firmly attaches itself in their place. When mercury replaces minerals and binds to these sites on a protein, it alters the protein's normal structure and function. As more and more mercury replaces these key minerals, the proteins will be less and less able to function properly.

Enzymes

Enzymes are also proteins, but they are generally smaller and have different functions. Every chemical reaction in the body requires a specific enzyme and every enzyme is necessary for optimal health. The body has over 3,000 kinds of enzymes and each one is made up of between 100 and 1,000 amino acids, in varying sequences. At any given time, a cell can contain many millions of enzymes (the number and kind depends on the cell's need for them).

Each enzyme is unique and each one is designed to carry out a specific function in an extraordinarily precise way, mainly by transporting substances, breaking down substances, or building them up. For example, table sugar (sucrose) is a disaccharide and is made up of two common monosaccharides—glucose and fructose. The enzyme sucrase is designed specifically to act as the key to open the lock that attaches these two monosaccharides together, freeing them to be used in other reactions. This lock-opening function is the sucrase enzyme's sole purpose—it doesn't take part in any other reaction. Other enzymes join together material needed to build or take apart cellular components, help repair damaged cells, and, on a larger scale, build muscle tissue.

Mercury has the same effect on enzymes as it does on proteins. When mercury attaches to a sulfur containing site on an enzyme, the enzyme will no longer work properly, or may not work at all. Trillions of reactions involving enzymes take place in the body every moment, and the proper function of all enzymes is crucial for optimal health. If one or two or 50 enzymes don't function correctly, it will be harmful on a cellular level, but may not be experienced as an observable symptom. But as mercury continues to alter or stop the critical enzymatic process, symptoms of chronic mercury poisoning will eventually appear.

Free Radical Generation

The direct effects of mercury on proteins and enzymes isn't the only damage it does to the body. Continuous exposure to mercury has an **indirect** effect by generating enormous amounts of free radicals. Any atom with at least one unpaired electron is called a free radical. Two of the most damaging free radicals are the superoxide radical and the hydroxyl radical. Because free radicals are highly reactive, they can participate in unwanted side reactions, resulting in cellular damage and making them a major contributor to degenerative diseases, heart disease, and cancer, to name but a few. Free radicals are also generated in cells during the normal process of cellular metabolism, such as the production of energy from food. Toxic substances, such as mercury pollutants, cigarette smoke, pesticides, and radiation can also generate huge amounts of free radicals.

Under normal conditions, the body has enough antioxidants available (particularly glutathione [GSH], alpha lipoic acid [ALA], vitamins C and E, selenium, and flavonoids) to neutralize free radicals. But if the production of free radicals becomes excessive, or antioxidant levels are low, extensive and long-term cellular damage can occur. Mercury is double trouble for the body because it not only generates huge numbers of free radicals but depletes GSH and ALA as they remove mercury from the body. In addition, the body now has the additional problem of removing, or safely storing, the minerals mercury has kicked off— zinc and copper. Both these minerals can be toxic in high amounts—and they can't be left floating around freely in a cell or the bloodstream. In high amounts, copper can lead to brain and liver damage and actually mimic some of mercury's symptoms, such as memory loss, fatigue, and headaches.

The Role of Glutathione (GSH) and
Alpha Lipoic Acid (ALA) in Removing Mercury from the Body

Removing mercury from the body is a very different process from how the body normally deals with other toxins. In effect, the body's antioxidants capture a toxin, transport it to the liver, and break it down into harmless, water-soluble substances that can easily be removed from the body via the detoxification pathways—feces, urine, lungs, hair, and skin. However, mercury in the body cannot be detoxified or broken down into anything except mercury. This means mercury must be physically removed, or escorted, if you will, from the body.

Both glutathione (GSH) and alpha lipoic acid (ALA) are heavy metal chelators, with GSH being the body's main mercury chelator. They find the mercury, pull it off from where it's attached to proteins and enzymes, carry it into liver, out through the common bile duct into the intestine, and out of the body via the feces. The consensus among researchers is that while it takes one molecule of ALA to remove one atom of mercury, it takes two molecules of GSH to effectively transport one atom of mercury out of the body.

The good news is that the body *can* remove mercury. It's amazingly intelligent and knows how toxic mercury is. So as long as it's able to, the body will remove millions of atoms of mercury daily. The bad news is that the process of removing mercury can create a serious deficiency in GSH and ALA. Of course both of these mercury chelators have other important functions, such as energy production and neutralizing free radicals. Both are manufactured by the body, but ALA is only produced in small amounts, and can be more rapidly depleted by mercury.

Mercury In Doesn't Mean Mercury Out

Another thing that makes mercury so toxic is the strong bond it forms with sulfhydryl group on proteins and enzymes. Glutathione (GSH) and alpha lipoic acid (ALA) are able to break that bond and safely escort mercury out of the body, but if the exposure to mercury is ongoing, these antioxidants will become seriously depleted over time. Bottom line—it may be easy for mercury to get into cells and easy to disrupt normal cellular function, but it isn't so easy to get mercury out.

If the amount of mercury coming in can be immediately removed, it won't cause any significant harm. But at some point, depending on the many factors we've already discussed, the incoming amount will surpass the body's ability to remove it, and mercury will begin to accumulate. At this point it's no longer mercury in, mercury out—it's mostly a lot of mercury in, and not much out.

A metaphor will be helpful here. Imagine your body as a factory full of workers called antioxidants, and there are two conveyor belts, one bringing containers of mercury in and the other carrying the containers out. The problem is that it takes two workers to carry each container of mercury out of the factory, and they can't get back in. This system will work well as long as the number of incoming containers is small and there are enough workers added to replace the ones who had to permanently leave. Under this scenario it would truly be mercury in and mercury out. But it doesn't take too much imagination to see what would happen if the amount of incoming mercury containers increased and no more workers could be found to replace those who left. In this case, all of the incoming mercury containers wouldn't be removed, and more and more would have to stay in the factory with no place to safely put them, thereby disrupting the system.

Glutathione (GSH) Loss Continues after Amalgam Removal

At first glance it would seem logical that once you remove the main source of mercury exposure (amalgam fillings), the problem will be solved. But this isn't how it works, and while I'll use glutathione as an example here, the same principles apply to alpha lipoic acid. By the time a person's amalgam fillings have been removed, most people will already be seriously deficient in GSH. Even after the fillings have been removed, if nothing is done to help the body rebuild its supply of GSH, more and more will be lost as the body continues its efforts to remove mercury. Over time, the net loss of glutathione means the body will progressively lose its ability to not only remove mercury and other heavy metals, but to adequately deal with the onslaught of free radicals and toxins. (Glutathione is also able to remove the other heavy metals, further depleting it.)

Given the poisonous nature of mercury, it's absolutely fantastic that the body can remove any of it. But the body was never designed to deal with the large, continuous amounts released by amalgam fillings, as well as other sources that didn't exist a few hundred years ago. Without a doubt, the damage the body sustains from mercury is bad news. But there's also good news. The human body is a miracle, and when it's provided the amino acids it needs to manufacture GSH and the other materials it needs to deal with mercury, it will be much more effective at removing what is stored and better able to protect itself from other harmful invaders. The concept of mercury detoxification is introduced in Chapter 11: "Mercury Detoxification."

The First Exposure to Mercury from Amalgam Fillings

I know this will surprise and shock you, but your first exposure to mercury from amalgam fillings can start long before they're ever put in your teeth. If your mother had amalgam fillings, your first exposure occurred at the moment of conception. Mercury also passes from mother to baby through breast milk. I'll discuss the detrimental effects of mercury on the fetus, nursing baby, and child in detail in Chapter 6, but I'm introducing it here because, when evaluating the health hazards of mercury fillings, you must understand that your exposure to mercury isn't just limited to your own amalgam fillings, eating contaminated fish, or your environmental and occupational exposure. Thus, the effects mercury can have on your body will ultimately be determined by your total exposure over time, including during fetal development and nursing.

Direct Effects of Mercury

Most sources of information dealing with chronic mercury poisoning only address the direct effects mercury has on the body. In the previous section I talked about some of the direct effects mercury has on proteins, hormones, enzymes, and DNA. These effects can contribute to many neurological issues, heart and kidney problems, chronic fatigue syndrome (CFS), and multiple sclerosis (MS), to name but a very few. Thousands of studies have been done that document mercury's negative impact on the body, and no scientist will dispute this information. (Chapter 5: "Symptoms and Diseases Related to Chronic Mercury Poisoning" has a comprehensive list of these effects.)

Scientists also know that mercury can interfere directly with disease-fighting white blood cells and can inactivate neutrophils, the most important type of white blood cell. White blood cells are essential components of the immune system and are responsible for killing bacteria inside the body and protecting it from infections.

Mercury's poisonous effects on the body are so widespread that estimates state that it can directly contribute to over 100 symptoms and diseases. The wide-ranging direct effects of mercury should never be overlooked or underestimated when assessing the total effect of mercury on your health. It's fair to say that you'll never be truly healthy as long as mercury vapor is being released from your amalgam fillings and mercury is still stored in your body.

Indirect Effects of Mercury

The indirect effects of mercury are primarily due to its ability to generate free radicals and its depleting effect on the body's most important mercury-removing antioxidants, GSH and ALA. There's no doubt that the combination of direct and indirect effects of mercury poisoning create a scenario far more damaging than the direct effects alone. The combination makes mercury a very potent and destructive two-edged sword. If mercury exposure continues over a long period of time, the indirect effects of mercury are at least as harmful, if not more so, than the direct effects.

In fact, indirect effects of chronic mercury poisoning can be compared to AIDS (Acquired Immune Deficiency Syndrome). HIV (Human Immunodeficiency Virus), the virus that causes AIDS, doesn't kill directly, but it can so weaken the immune system that it no longer has the ability to protect itself against the onslaught of heavy metals, toxins, bacteria, and other harmful substances. Thus, people with AIDS don't die of AIDS, they die of pneumonia, cancer, kidney failure, etc. But the fact that HIV itself isn't the direct cause of death doesn't make it any less lethal.

Chronic exposure to mercury may not be as devastating, but the analogy is accurate in that given enough time, mercury can dramatically inhibit the function of the immune system, opening the door to other serious health problems. Of course, the fact that both AIDS and chronic mercury poisoning significantly depress the immune system makes it imperative for anyone with HIV or AIDS to safely have their amalgam fillings removed and replaced with a safe alternative as soon as possible.

When Mercury Accumulates

As you've learned, it can take months to many years for the body to accumulate enough mercury to cause a symptom related to chronic mercury poisoning. But even if you've not yet exhibited any related symptoms, it doesn't mean the mercury isn't doing any damage. For example, say that the body didn't exhibit a mercury related symptom until 13 mcg of mercury accumulated in a particular part. Does that mean the first 12 mcg of accumulated mercury was harmless? The answer is an emphatic *no*! Every atom of mercury is poisonous, not just the last one.

That old parable of the straw breaking the camel's back effectively demonstrates this point—just think of your body as the camel, each straw as a small amount of mercury entering the body, and the farmer as an amalgam filling. In this modified parable, the farmer loads straw after straw on his camel's back. Finally, the farmer feels he has added as much straw as the camel can carry. But then he sees a single straw lying on the ground. "Why not?" he says. "My camel is strong enough to carry just one extra piece of straw!" But when he adds the last straw, it breaks the camel's back.

Of course it wasn't the last straw, or the last single microgram of mercury, that broke the camel's back—it's the total of all the straws, or all the atoms, including the first and the last and all the ones in between. Over time, if the source of mercury isn't removed, the majority of people exposed to it will have to deal with the "last straw." Sadly, it doesn't end at the last straw. As more and more mercury accumulates, more and more symptoms directly and indirectly related to chronic mercury poisoning will appear, and get worse over time. The key to understanding everything so far, and what the next chapter will discuss, hinges on you keeping in mind that there is no safe level of mercury. Every atom is toxic, and it can never be considered harmless.

What Have You Learned?

You know now that if you have amalgam fillings, you are mercury toxic to some degree. And mercury can be a contributing factor to every symptom or health problem you may have. You've learned that as long as your body is still being poisoned by mercury, you can never achieve optimal health.

The fact is, the symptoms you're experiencing that are related to mercury poisoning will not improve until the fillings are removed. Only then can your body begin to deal with the stored mercury. Studies show that some improvement in symptoms will take place over time once the amalgams are removed. But to accelerate and maximize symptom improvement, most people will need a detoxification program (see Chapter 11: "Mercury Detoxification"). Thus, removing the source of mercury is a critical and an absolutely necessary first step. But it isn't the only step.

What's Next?

Now that you know how mercury does its damage, it's important to know how mercury affects your health. The next chapter will list the many symptoms and diseases directly or indirectly related to chronic mercury poisoning. It will also discuss mercury allergies and mercury's relationship to autoimmune diseases.

Five

Symptoms and Diseases Related to Chronic Mercury Poisoning

There are thousands of scientific studies showing that chronic mercury poisoning can contribute to over 100 symptoms and diseases. Combined with its indirect effects, mercury will, to some degree, negatively affect every aspect of your health.

In general, the effect of mercury released from amalgams on your overall health—particularly the health of your immune system—will depend on these factors:

- how many fillings you have, or had
- type of amalgam, high or low copper content
- how long you've had them
- how they're stimulated
- how often they're stimulated
- how long the stimulation lasts
- your exposure to other forms of mercury
- the total amount of mercury you've been exposed to in your life, including during fetal development
- the amount still present in your body after amalgam removal

Emotional and Psychological Effects of Mercury

Not only does mercury have an impact on your physical health, it has an impact on your mental health as well. Mercury is classified as a neurotoxin, a toxin that specifically targets nerve cells. As such, it can also cause or contribute to emotional and psychological issues, such as depression, anxiety, mood swings, and memory loss. I can't stress enough the importance of this fact. Most people I've consulted with over the years believed mercury only had an impact on their physical health—such as chronic fatigue, tremors, and heart issues.

As you'll see in the "Emotions" section of the chart on the next page, mercury can cause or contribute to a number of a very common emotional/psychological problems. This isn't to say mercury is the ony cause, but if a person with any of these symptoms has amalgam fillings, mercury has to be considered a significant contributor. In fact, most of the psychologists, psychiatrists, and counselors I've spoken to were quite surprised to discover that mercury could play such a major role in the emotional and psychological health of their patients.

Chronic Mercury Poisoning and Related Diseases

Chronic mercury poisoning has also been directly connected to the following diseases and health problems. But again, mercury's indirect effects could make this list much, much longer.

Chronic Mercury Poisoning: Related Diseases	
Acrodynia	Emphysema
Alzheimer's	Fibromyalgia
Anterior Lateral Sclerosis (ALS)	Hormonal Dysfunction
Asthma	Intestinal Dysfunction
Arthritis	Immune System Disorders
Autism	Kidney Disease
Autoimmune Diseases	Learning Disorders
Candida	Liver Disorders
Cardiovascular Disease	Lupus
Chronic Fatigue Syndrome	Metabolic Encephalopathy
Crohn's Disease	Multiple Sclerosis (MS)
Depression	Reproductive Disorders
Developmental Defects	Parkinson's Disease
Diabetes	Senile Dementia
Eczema	Thyroid Disease

Common Symptoms of Chronic Mercury Poisoning

The following chart lists some of the common symptoms directly related to chronic mercury poisoning. But remember that mercury can indirectly cause great harm by depleting antioxidants and lowering the body's resistance to other diseases. Therefore, if you have amalgam fillings and have a health issue you don't see listed, it doesn't mean mercury isn't contributing to it or making it worse.

Common Symptoms of Chronic Mercury Poisoning	
Type	*Symptoms*
Digestive System	Colitis Diarrhea/Constipation Loss of Appetite Weight Loss Nausea/Vomiting
Emotions	Aggressiveness Anger Anxiety Confusion Depression Fear/Nervousness Hallucination Lethargy Manic Depression Mood Swings Shyness
Energy Levels	Apathy Chronic Fatigue Restlessness
Head	Dizziness Faintness Headaches (frequent) Ringing in Ears
Heart	Anemia Chest Pain Heartbeat, Rapid or Irregular
Lungs	Asthma/Bronchitis Chest Congestion Shallow Respiration Shortness of Breath
Muscles & Joints	Cramping Joint Aches Muscle Aches Muscle Weakness Stiffness
Neurological/ Mental	Fine Tremor Lack of Concentration Learning Disorders Memory Loss, Short and Long Term Numbness Slurred Speech
Nose	Inflammation of the Nose Sinusitis Excessive Mucus Formation Stuffy Nose
Oral/Throat	Bad Breath (halitosis) Bone Loss Burning Sensation Chronic Coughing Gingivitis/Bleeding Gums Inflammation of the Gums Leukoplakia (white patches) Metallic Taste Mouth Inflammation Sore Throat Ulcers of Oral Cavity

Common Symptoms of Chronic Mercury Poisoning	
Type	*Symptoms*
Other	Allergies Anorexia Excessive Blushing Genital Discharge Gland Swelling Hair Loss Hypoxia Illnesses (frequent) Insomnia Loss of Sense of Smell Perspiration (excessive) Renal Failure Skin Cold and Clammy Skin Problems Vision Problems (tunnel vision) Water Retention (edema)

Other Factors

When it comes to establishing the causative link between the symptoms and diseases related to chronic mercury poisoning, it's important to also consider other contributing factors. For example, genetics, poor diet, abusive lifestyle, toxic environment, occupational exposure, and substance abuse—either alone or in combination—can play significant roles.

In fact, the risk of developing a health problem related to chronic mercury poisoning can significantly increase when these other factors *and* mercury are present together. While there's no doubt that mercury poisoning is a contributor to every health issue, it isn't the only one to be concerned about.

A Triple-Edged Sword: Allergies and Mercury

You've seen how the direct and indirect effects of mercury make it a double-edged health hazard. But if you're allergic to mercury, a third edge has to be added to mercury's destructive sword. Generally, an allergy occurs when you are exposed to an allergen in the environment—pollutants, allergenic products, plants, and food substances. Once identified, most of those sources can be eliminated or controlled.

For example, if you discover that you have a wheat allergy, you can immediately eliminate it from your diet. But if you're sensitive to mercury from amalgam fillings, the mercury allergen won't go away unless you remove the fillings. Until then, you will be exposed to this allergen every minute of every hour of every day . . . even when the fillings aren't stimulated. (Even though mercury vapor won't be released from an amalgam filling at room temperature, the temperature of the mouth, as you know from taking your temperature, is a tad over 98° F/37° C. At this temperature small amounts of mercury will be released even if the fillings are not stimulated.)

Another important aspect of an allergic response is the extent of exposure, which in turn determines the severity of the reaction. For example, you could be allergic to ragweed pollen and hardly notice it if you breathed in only a few grains. But if someone shook the weed in your face, exposing you to millions of grains, you'd have a much more serious reaction.

Similarly, if you have only one amalgam filling that isn't being constantly stimulated and a reasonably well-functioning immune system, your allergic response could be tolerable, with low-grade symptoms. Most likely it wouldn't dramatically affect the quality of your life. But if you had 12 amalgam fillings, chewed gum, ground your teeth, and snacked often, your body's response to the mercury allergen would be far more intense.

Continuous exposure to an allergen will also significantly stress your immune system. But few people think of their fillings and the mercury they release as a cause or contributor to allergies. Fewer still have been advised to be tested for an allergy to mercury. The effects on your health of an ongoing allergy to mercury would be bad enough, but remember, you'd also have to add the harm caused by the direct and indirect effects of it. The good news is that there's an excellent test available to determine if you're allergic to mercury. The MELISA® (Memory Lymphocyte Immuno Stimulation Assay) test, invented by Profesor Vera Stejskal, is the world's leading test for hypersensitivity to metals. Refer to Appendix A for more information about this test.

The ADA and Mercury Allergy

In 1984 the ADA actually admitted what it had adamantly denied for over 150 years—amalgam fillings release mercury vapor. But instead of banning them, the ADA shifted its position and said that although amalgam fillings release small amounts of mercury, it isn't enough to harm anyone, *except those with an allergy to mercury.*

In that same year, the ADA stated in an article in *Science Digest* that 5 percent of the total population of the U.S. was allergic to mercury. That figure wouldn't be significant if no one had mercury amalgam fillings. But in 1984 over 100 million people in the U.S. had amalgam fillings. So all of a sudden 5 percent becomes very significant number. That figure—straight from the ADA—meant that 5 million people were allergic to the mercury in their fillings.

Of course, an allergy is technically classified as a medical problem and can be very serious, even fatal. Thus, for the ADA to admit that 5 million people would have an identifiable medical problem directly related to the mercury released from their amalgam fillings was amazing, considering that the ADA insists that amalgam fillings aren't hazardous to your health.

Well, someone in the organization must have figured out that 5 million didn't sound so good, and the ADA quickly re-evaluated its position. Suddenly they claimed it was 3 percent, but gave no explanation as to why and didn't cite any studies to support it. Again, that percentage may not sound so bad, but it still meant that 3 million people with amalgam fillings would be allergic to mercury. Apparently even *that* figure didn't sit well with the ADA, so soon after, it arbitrarily lowered it to 1 percent of the population.

But even 1 percent wasn't low enough. According to an article in the ADA's official publication, the *Journal of the American Dental Association* (2003), it referred to a study conducted by French researchers that found only 41 published cases, from 1905 to 1986, of allergic reactions to mercury from amalgam fillings—in the entire world. Based on that, the ADA now says that less than 50 people are allergic to mercury!

Whew! Trying to keep up with the ADA and their ongoing defense of mercury fillings can be exhausting. But as you'll soon see, others take a much different view of the mercury allergy issue.

Other Sources of Information

Fortunately, the ADA isn't the only source of information about the percentage of people who are allergic to mercury. Other estimates range from 1 to 35 percent, with some going even higher. Today those numbers would correspond to between 1.5 and 52 million Americans suffering from a mercury allergy. These percentages aren't small by anyone's standards. Yet percentages only yield numbers and not names. So your concern should be discovering whether you're one of the millions who are allergic to mercury.

To be honest, I don't believe anyone really knows exactly how many people have amalgam fillings, or how many of those who do will be allergic to the mercury released from them. We do know that millions of people have allergies, and that number is increasing dramatically. One study by S.J. Arbes et al showed that nearly 55 percent of Americans suffer from one or more allergens. Another study was conducted with fourth-year dental students, and it showed that 44 percent of them were allergic to mercury.

We also know that billions of dollars are spent every year on allergy treatment and medicine. Based on my research, I believe the reason more and more people are suffering from allergies is because we are being bombarded by more toxins and allergens than ever before. The depletion of antioxidants by chronic exposure to mercury from amalgam fillings has caused our immune system to become overwhelmed.

Mercury: The Hidden Allergy

When confronted with a patient who exhibits allergy symptoms, health professionals usually focus on food, the environment, and industrial pollutants as probable causes. Until recently, the medical profession, holistic or traditional, hasn't spent much time looking at mercury as one of the sources. There is a very high incidence of oral contact dermatitis for those with amalgam fillings, and contact dermatitis is classified as a skin allergy. I also believe that many of the symptoms of mercury allergy are strikingly similar to those of multiple sclerosis (MS), chronic fatigue syndrome (CFS), and other autoimmune diseases.

When an amalgam filling is stimulated, elemental mercury will puddle on the surface of it, and both the elemental mercury and its vapor will come in direct contact with the skin, particularly the gum and cheek mucosa tissue closest to the filling. Remember, regulatory agencies recommend not touching mercury and I'm sure that also means not having it touch you.

A 2003 study of 189 patients showed that 80 percent of those with lesions next to amalgam fillings were allergic to the mercury in the filling. If 80 percent of those with amalgam fillings developed contact dermatitis, that would work out to around 120 million people in the U.S. alone—a significantly greater number than the ADA's 41 cases.

In another study by Finne et al, 29 patients with oral lichen planus and amalgam fillings were patch tested for contact allergy to dental materials. (Oral lichen planus is a chronic inflammatory disease that causes a rash on the tissue lining the mouth, tongue, and gums, which some consider an autoimmune disease.) Eighteen of these patients (62 percent) had a contact allergy to mercury. In a control group, the frequency of mercury allergy was 3.2 percent. In four of the patients, all the amalgam restorations were removed and replaced by gold and composite materials. The lesions healed completely in three of these patients after an observation period of one year, and the remaining case showed considerable improvement.

In a smaller study by Pang et al, 19 patients had oral lichenoid lesions (a common lesion of the mouth) in close contact with their mercury fillings. All showed positive patch tests for mercury compounds. Sixteen patients had their amalgam fillings replaced, and in 13 of them the lesions completely healed and one showed marked improvement. This works out to 87 percent cured or show-ing significant improvement after amalgam removal. The study concluded that oral lichenoid lesions can be caused by mercury released from amalgam fillings and can be effectively treated by having the fillings removed.

In another study by Henrik Lichtenberg, 65 of the participants had allergy symptoms. When their amalgams were removed, 40 showed a marked improvement and 3 were completely free of their allergy symptoms, or 66 percent improved or were cured. (See more on the Lichtenberg study in Chapter 12: "Health Improve-ments Related to Amalgam Removal and Mercury Detoxification.")

Thankfully, more health professionals—especially those who focus their practices on allergies and dermatology—are beginning to realize that mercury is a common allergen. It's not really surprising, given the fact that over 150 million Americans have amalgam fillings and the mercury they release comes in direct and constant contact with the tissue of the mouth. Given the large number of people with amalgams, allergies to mercury must be taken into consideration when searching out the source of an allergen.

In over 30 years as a mercury free dentist, I've seen many people show imme-diate improvement in their allergy symptoms after the safe removal and replace-ment of amalgam fillings. And as you've seen, the preceding studies show that mercury allergies are common—not rare as the ADA contends.

Autoimmune Disease and Mercury

Here's another little-known fact about mercury and allergies: mercury can trigger autoimmune diseases. Autoimmune diseases are a very serious type of immune response (allergic reaction), and there are over 60 recognized ones, affecting nearly 10 million people in the U.S. alone.

These diseases include multiple sclerosis (MS), rheumatoid arthritis, lupus, Addison's disease, Crohn's disease, and myasthenia gravis. (You'll find a more complete list of autoimmune diseases later in this chapter.) There are approxi-mately 20 more diseases or syndromes that are thought to be autoimmune diseases and could be related to mercury exposure, including chronic fatigue syndrome, psoriasis, and scleroderma.

Autoimmune disease occurs when the body produces an immunological, or allergic, reaction to itself. This reaction happens when a protein has been so altered by mercury, or other substances, that the body's lymphocytes, a type of white blood cell that recognize a protein as a friend or foe, no longer recognizes the mercury-altered protein as a friend. If lymphocytes indentify a foe, they attack it and literally break it apart, resulting in an inflammatory response.

Mercury's role in autoimmune disease is a classic example of its indirect effect on the body, and there's no doubt that mercury at least acts as a major contributor to this very serious health issue. Yet despite overwhelming evidence of its role, the ADA totally discounts mercury as a factor in autoimmune disease.

The ADA has assumed the right to state its case about amalgams but, in my opinion, it doesn't have the right to speak for medical doctors and other health professionals about *any* medical issue related to chronic mercury poisoning. After all, the diagnosis and treatment of allergies are medical issues, not dental ones. I doubt very much that you would even consider going to a dentist to diagnose or treat an allergy. (Of course, when the cause is diagnosed as mercury from dental fillings, the mercury safe dentist will play a contributing role by safely removing them.)

Testing for Mercury Allergy and Amalgam Removal

If you have allergic reactions or related health symptoms for which your health professional can't find a specific cause, have him or her test you for an allergy to mercury. If it turns out you're allergic to mercury and have amalgam fillings, you have a pretty good idea of what you should do about it.

But determining whether or not you're allergic to mercury takes on greater importance when it comes to removing your amalgam fillings. If you're allergic to mercury and don't have your fillings removed in a safe way, you'll be exposed to extraordinarily high amounts of mercury vapor—amounts that could trigger an even more severe allergic reaction. I believe that those who have the greatest negative response to unsafe amalgam removal are those who are allergic to mercury.

As amazing as it may sound, in my 30 years as a mercury free and mercury safe dentist, I've never heard of a pro-amalgam dentist recommending that a patient be tested for an allergy to mercury—even though the ADA has agreed that mercury is an allergen.

Signs and Symptoms of Mercury Allergy

Testing is the best way to accurately diagnose an allergy to mercury, but you can also watch out for these signs and symptoms:

- unusual reactions to the placement or removal of mercury fillings
- feeling exhausted soon after the placement or removal of mercury fillings
- inability to function normally after the placement or removal of mercury fillings

- sores or unusual lesions on the inside of your mouth, especially in the area close to mercury fillings, or in the area close to a gold crown. (This happens because mercury will not only be in contact with the tissue closest to an amalgam, but will migrate from the amalgam to the gold crown and deposit in the gum tissue around it.)

The following table lists some of the more common symptoms of an allergy. Again, these symptoms are generalized indications of an allergy. They have more meaning if they appear or increase in severity during the placement or unsafe removal of mercury fillings. If you're unsure about the source of your symptoms, check with an allergy specialist—and I don't mean your pro-amalgam dentist. A reliable way to test for a mercury allergy is to take the MELISA® test, which measures hypersensitivity to a number of metals, including mercury. You'll find information about this test in Appendix A.

Allergy Symptoms	
Absentmindedness	Joint Aches and Pains
Breathing Difficulties	Muscle Pain
Burning Eyes	Nasal Congestion
Concentration Difficulties	Nausea
Cough	Postnasal Drip
Depression	Rapid Pulse
Diarrhea	Smell Impairment
Dizziness	Skin Rashes
Ear Ringing	Sleeping Difficulties
Flushing	Sneezing
Headaches	Swallowing Difficulties
Heart Palpitations	Swelling
Hives	Throat Irritation, Itching
Irritability	Tiredness
Itchy, Runny, or Tingling Nose	Vomiting
Itchy, Watery, Crusty, Red Eyes	Wheezing

Partial List of Symptoms and Diseases Related to Autoimmune Disease	
Addison's Disease	Lupus Erythematosis (LE)
Aplastic Anemia	Multiple Chemical Sensitivity (MCS)
Autoimmune Hepatitis	Multiple Sclerosis (MS)
Celiac Disease	Myalgic Encephalitis (ME)
Chronic Fatigue Syndrome (CFS)	Myasthenia Gravis

Partial List of Symptoms and Diseases Related to Autoimmune Disease	
Crohn's Disease	Oral Burning and Itching
Diabetes Mellitus, Type 1	Oral Lichen Planus (OLP)
Food Allergies (unexplained)	Ord's Thyroiditis
Fibromyalgia	Pemphigus
Graves' Disease	Pernicious Anemia
Guillain-Barré Syndrome (GBS)	Rheumatoid Arthritis (RA)
Hashimoto's Disease	Sjogren's Syndrome
Immune-Mediated Pathology	Skin Diseases such as Eczema or Psoriasis

Mercury Allergy and its Relationship to Disease

Being allergic to mercury is bad enough, but research done by MELISA® shows that the existence of any allergy to metals, including mercury, can aggravate the diseases listed in the preceding chart.

No Such Thing as Harmless Mercury

After reviewing all the mercury-related symptoms, diseases, and disorders, you can understand why the World Health Organization (WHO) states that there's no safe or harmless level of mercury. Even if the harmful effects of mercury were limited to its relationship to allergies, it would still be a major health concern for tens of millions of people.

Scientifically, medically, logically, and legally, the term "harmless" can never be used to describe mercury. Think about it in terms of smoking. Smoking a few cigarettes daily may not kill you, or even make you sick. But smoking a few can't be considered *harmless*, even if you don't ultimately get cancer or a related respiratory disease. The fact is that even those few cigarettes still compromise your health to some degree. For a person in poor health, a few cigarettes a day could be even more disastrous than to someone who is in good health. The same is true for mercury exposure. A person in poor health with just a few amalgams will have an increased risk of developing symptoms of chronic mercury poisoning than a healthy person with the same number of fillings.

When dealing with any poison, everything is relative to its toxicity, the size of the dose, how often it's taken, and the person's overall health. For example, if you only have one or two amalgam fillings and don't grind your teeth, your risk factor is significantly lower than if you have 12 amalgams and grind your teeth. What makes the mercury vapor released from amalgam fillings so toxic is that, unlike other sources of exposure, this powerful poison is *continuously* released into the body.

Something to Think About

The bottom line is that if you have, or had, amalgam (silver) fillings, you are mercury toxic to some degree, and your immune system will have been harmed. If you have any of the related symptoms or diseases listed in this chapter, are prone to allergies, or have a compromised immune system, you should seriously consider having your toxic fillings safely removed and replaced with a safe dental restoration. I also believe participation in a safe and effective mercury detoxification program would be very beneficial on many levels. Another book I've written, *Mercury Detoxification: The Natural Way to Remove Mercury from Your Body,* will guide you through every step of the mercury detoxification process. The book is available on my website, www.dentalwellness4u.com.

What's Next?

We've covered a lot of ground, and hopefully you know much more about this subject than when you opened the book. But we're not finished, and I consider the next chapter—about the effects of mercury from amalgam fillings on the fetus, nursing baby, and child—to be one of, if not *the,* most important chapter in this book.

Six

The Effects of Mercury on the Fetus, Nursing Baby, and Child

A **child's first exposure** to mercury from amalgam fillings can occur *at the moment of conception!* If the mother has mercury amalgam (silver) fillings in her teeth, the fetus will not only be exposed to mercury released from its mother's fillings at the moment of its conception, but throughout the entire gestation period. Think about that and the implications it holds! This means the fetus is being exposed to poisonous elemental mercury from dental fillings before it even has a tooth! Everything I discuss in this chapter is related to this important fact.

Many people are aware that mercury from thimerosal (the preservative used in vaccinations) and genetics have been suggested as the primary causes of autism and other learning and developmental disorders. But as I'll explain later in this chapter, neither genetics nor mercury from vaccinations can account for the high incidence of autism in our population today. Based on my research, the most significant factor in the cause of autism and other learning and developmental disorders—which has remained hidden until now—is mercury released from amalgam fillings. This is the key to understanding how destructive mercury is to the fetus and nursing baby.

In this chapter I'll also talk about solutions and how you can minimize the risk of having a child with a learning or developmental disorder by having your mercury amalgam fillings safely removed prior to conception. It's my sincere hope that the information found in this chapter will encourage women of child-bearing age to have these toxic fillings safely removed prior to becoming pregnant, and to then participate in a mercury detoxification program. If this isn't possible, see Chapter 10: "Reducing Mercury Exposure from Amalgam (Silver) Fillings" which offers suggestions to minimize your exposure to mercury from the amalgam fillings you still have in your teeth. But first let's start with what we know and then I'll connect the dots.

The Relationship of Mercury to Neurological Development

As you know, mercury poses a serious health risk for adults, but the mercury vapor released from amalgam (silver) fillings is infinitely more toxic to the fetus and nursing baby. For example, mercury is known to cause birth defects and learning and developmental disorders. What you'll learn here will be an eye-opener, and no objective book on amalgam fillings can be considered complete or accurate without discussing this extremely important subject.

Exposure to mercury during early neurological development can cause or contribute to every type of learning or developmental disorder. Autism is on the rise—in 2007 the Centers for Disease Control (CDC) estimated that one out of 150 children born in the U.S. is diagnosed with autism. This is an 800 percent increase since the early 1990s. I'll focus on autism in this chapter because it's the best known, and most studied, type of learning and developmental disorder. Studies have proven that mercury can:

- cause or contribute to autism, or any other infant or childhood learning or developmental disorder

- negatively effect, both short and long term, the immune system of the baby and child

- contribute to a range of other health issues in infancy, early childhood, and as an adult

Many learning and developmental disorders and syndromes have been labeled, such as autism, Asperger syndrome, attention deficit disorder (ADD), and obsessive compulsive disorder (OCD). But what we know is just the tip of the iceberg, and organizing the various symptoms into categories isn't easy. For example, a child may exhibit symptoms associated with a number of different learning and developmental disorders, making it difficult to place him or her into any specific group.

Thus, many of these disorders have been lumped under a much larger umbrella, such as pervasive developmental disorders (PDD). PDD specifically refers to five disorders, all of which show, to varying degrees, delays in developing normal communication skills, repetitive patterns, and social interactions. Autism is the most well known of the PDDs and is also referred to as autism spectrum disorder. The four other PDDs are:

- Asperger syndrome

- childhood disintegrative disorder (CDD)

- Rett syndrome

- pervasive developmental disorder not otherwise specified (PDD-NOS)

While the numerous symptoms related to autism have been defined, determining a specific cause has eluded researchers. If the origin of a disease or health issue can't be proven, it's referred to as being idiopathic, meaning it occurs spontaneously or its cause is unknown. This lack of a specific origin opens a Pandora's Box of possibilities and allows many opinions and theories to compete with each other. For the many reasons I'll present, I've chosen mercury as the main causative agent, primarily the mercury released from amalgam fillings.

The Relationship of Chronic Mercury Poisoning to Autism

Autism is a neurological disorder, and nearly every associated symptom closely correlates to those of chronic mercury poisoning. Understanding the relationship between autism and chronic mercury poisoning will shed new light on this subject. I've extensively researched chronic mercury poisoning since 1996 and have found the similarities to autism extraordinarily revealing. In fact, chronic mercury poisoning and autism share many comparable symptoms. In my opinion, this comparison alone provides enough evidence to suggest that continuous exposure to mercury during fetal development is a major factor in autism.

A comparison chart from the brilliant work of autism researchers Sallie Bernard et al, compares the specific symptoms of chronic mercury poisoning that are exhibited at a young age with the known symptoms of autism. This chart compared 15 specific traits associated with autism—such as speech, language, hearing, and motor disorders—with those exhibited by mercury poisoning. The symptoms exhibited by each group are nearly identical.

The chart is extensive, and for those interested in the subject, it's a must-see. You can access it by going to my website, www.dentalwellness4u.com, and clicking on the "Autism" link in the Frequently Asked Questions (FAQ) menu on the homepage. Alternately, you can visit the website listed at the end of this chapter to view the chart and access more in-depth information regarding the relationship of autism to mercury from vaccinations. Sallie Bernard's group has done a tremendous job of educating the public about autism. Information about how to contact them is also found at the end of this chapter.

Genetics and Vaccinations

Genetics

To date, those who refuse to acknowledge the role of vaccinations in causing autism believe genetics is the major contributor. For a long time, genetics has been a convenient scapegoat, or catchall, and while it certainly could be *one* of the causes, genetics alone will *never* account for the high incidence of autism in our population today. The role mercury plays in causing genetic mutations, particularly during fetal development, *must* also be considered alongside genetics.

Mercury is classified as a "mutagenic" substance and is also known to be "teratogenic." A mutagenic substance is any agent that causes a permanent change in genetic material, resulting in a mutation. Mutations can cause birth defects and learning and developmental disorders. A teratogenic substance is anything that disrupts the growth and development of the embryo and fetus, leading to neurological and central nervous system disorders.

It logically follows that any exposure to mercury during fetal development could play a significant role in the genetic mutations that result in autism and other learning and developmental disorders. Even the constant 2 percent mutation rate in nature (where that same mutation rate will appear without any known reason or cause) does not account for the huge increase in autism. Of course there are other causes of genetic mutations, such as radiation, ultraviolet light, viruses, and numerous chemicals. A genetic flaw can also be inherited.

When autism was first diagnosed as a unique disorder in the 1940s, it was considered a rare occurrence. Then, starting in the early 1990s, diagnosed cases of autism in the U.S. increased dramatically. The number of school-age children who were diagnosed with it increased by over 800 percent. Scientists know that on its own, genetics cannot sufficiently account for that huge increase. (I personally believe that the introduction of high copper, non-gamma 2 amalgams in the late 1960s and early 1970s played a significant role in this increase.)

Vaccinations

Many autism organizations believe vaccinations to be the major cause of autism. Actually, it's not the vaccine itself that's the guilty party, but organic ethylmercury found in the preservative thimerosal, which contains up to 50 percent organic ethylmercury. While early exposure to acute doses of mercury from vaccinations is no doubt a contributing factor in autism, vaccinations alone can't account for the huge rise in autism. For example, there are those who suffer from autism who have never been vaccinated. And there are also those who were given the full range of vaccinations and didn't develop autism.

If both genetics and vaccinations can be ruled out as the primary cause of autism, then what can we attribute it to? Although there could be a number of independent causes of autism, such as inherited genes, I offer a more realistic theory—mercury from amalgam fillings. As you'll see, this theory goes much farther toward solving the mystery.

Think about this for a moment. No one advocates exposing the fetus or nursing baby to any toxin or poison and many laws and regulations are in place to protect them from such exposure. Yet if the mother has amalgam fillings, the fetus could be exposed to amounts of mercury that regulatory agencies wouldn't allow an adult to be exposed to!

First Exposure: Where It All Begins

Although I introduced this concept at the beginning of the chapter, it is so important that it deserves to be repeated. **A person's first exposure to mercury from amalgam fillings occurs at the moment of conception.** If the mother has amalgam (silver) fillings in her teeth, the fetus will be exposed to mercury released from them at the moment of conception and throughout the entire gestation period. The bad news doesn't end there. If the nursing mother has amalgam fillings, the child will also be exposed to mercury released from those fillings for as long as the child is being nursed. The nursing period is a critically important developmental time for the child, both physically and neurologically—and mercury passes into breast milk and on to the nursing baby. One study showed that 5 percent of the mercury a mother who is nursing her baby excretes is via breast milk. Others feel that figure is higher.

Let's not forget that the fetus and nursing baby can also receive mercury from other sources that the mother is exposed to, particularly contaminated fish. But while those sources can't be ignored, they don't represent the same kind of 24/7 exposure that amalgam fillings do.

In addition to the continuous exposure to mercury from amalgam fillings, most babies in modernized countries could receive up to 23 vaccinations by age two, with the first immunization given at birth. If thimerosal is used as a preservative in these vaccinations, each shot will contain approximately 237 mcg of highly toxic ethylmercury—with some children receiving up to six vaccinations during one visit to the doctor. Such a large dose of mercury so soon after birth makes it easy to understand how mercury from vaccinations could be a contributing factor to learning and developmental disorders and other health issues. But what must be understood about this relationship is that *a child will have already been exposed to significant amounts of mercury from the mother's amalgam fillings for nine months before even receiving that first vaccination!*

Exposure to significant amounts of mercury during development can be extremely harmful to the fetus. When you combine continuous fetal exposure to mercury from amalgams with exposure to organic mercury from vaccinations, as well as what the baby receives when he or she nurses, the impact will be significantly amplified. But while my research indicates mercury from amalgams plays a key role in the cause of autism, it isn't productive to focus on a single source of mercury as the sole causative factor, given the number of mercury variables.

For example, you could argue that the fetus received so much mercury from its mother's amalgam fillings that this amount alone could cause autism. Or you could argue that the amount received during fetal development wasn't enough to cause autism, but adding mercury from vaccinations tipped the scale. Another combination could be that the fetus received so much mercury from its mother's fillings and more from nursing that it would still develop autism, without being vaccinated. *But the most potent combination of all is a child being exposed to large amounts of elemental mercury as a fetus and during nursing, and then to mercury from the full complement of vaccinations.*

Amount of Exposure to the Fetus and Baby

The range of learning and developmental disorders varies widely from mild to severe. Because a mother, and therefore the fetus and nursing baby, could receive mercury from many sources, each must be taken into consideration. But the source of mercury is only one factor, and the timing, amount, and duration of exposure will play critical roles.

For example, one mother had only two small amalgams during the period the fetus was developing. Another mother had 12, ground her teeth, and had some old amalgams replaced with new amalgams during this period. When the two examples are compared, it's easy to see that the fetus in the second example will be exposed to much higher amounts of mercury than the former.

Variations can also occur in regards to nursing. For example, the woman with only two amalgams did not nurse her baby, but the mother with 12 amalgams nursed for two years. In addition, the number of vaccinations must also be factored in when considering the amount of mercury received during the critical first years of development. The mother with only two amalgams did not have her baby immunized, whereas the baby from the mother with 12 amalgams had the full complement of vaccinations.

These examples cover a wide range of possibilities, but they're not extreme and the possible combinations are endless. The amount of mercury the fetus and nursing baby are exposed to, and when the exposure took place, will vary greatly, and this could also account for the wide range of symptoms and the different degrees in severity of autism.

The important point here is that a clear connection exists between the fetus and nursing baby and the extent of early exposure to mercury from amalgam fillings. So even though all other sources of mercury can't be eliminated as participants in causing autism, I consider mercury from the mother's fillings the dominant factor.

The most important aspects of neurological development take place during fetal development, and it's during this period that the fetus is most vulnerable to mercury. Autism researchers suggest that during the early stage of fetal development it only takes a relatively small amount of mercury to cause or contribute to a number of birth defects, including learning and developmental disorders. One study by Mahafey and Rice showed that if a mother was exposed to mercury during pregnancy, the newborn baby's mercury levels could be from 30 to 100 percent higher than the mother's!

Remember that the child's early exposure to mercury doesn't end with nursing and vaccinations. The majority of children will also be exposed to mercury from their own amalgam fillings, beginning with their baby teeth as early as age two. By age two to three, the initial symptoms of autism will have appeared, but it's possible that this additional exposure to mercury the baby received from his or her own amalgams could make the symptoms of autism even worse.

Understanding Why Mercury is So Poisonous to the Fetus and Nursing Baby

The key to understanding this is to recognize that when the mother is exposed to elemental mercury vapor, the fetus and baby are too. But what makes it much, much worse is that the fetus doesn't have its own immune system, or a blood-brain barrier, nor can it eliminate mercury. In short, the fetus has no protection against mercury.

A baby's immune system doesn't fully develop for at least one month after he or she is born. Prior to this time, the baby relies on the mother's immune system to provide protection from bacteria, toxins, free radicals, and mercury. The problem is that the immune system of a mother with amalgam fillings will already be compromised to some degree, and it won't be nearly as effective at protecting the fetus.

The Many Factors Involved in Fetal Exposure to Mercury from Amalgams

We know that the fetus is extraordinarily susceptible to any mutagenic substance. Mercury is high on that list and, as previously discussed, its effect on the fetus will be dependent on the extent of the mother's exposure. You can refer back to Chapters 3 and 4 for a full discussion of the factors determining the degree and duration of exposure, but here's a brief review:

- how many amalgam fillings the mother has

- the type of amalgam, high or low copper content

- how large the fillings are

- how long the fillings have been in place

- how the fillings are stimulated

- how long they are stimulated

- how often they are stimulated

- the health of the mother's immune system

Another important factor to consider is whether or not the mother had any of her old amalgam fillings removed and replaced with new amalgams while she was pregnant or nursing. Or if she had any new amalgam fillings put in during this period. The greatest exposure to mercury, for those with amalgams, occurs when they are placed and removed. So this means that the greatest exposure to the fetus and nursing baby also takes place during those times. This acute dose of mercury, coming at a critical period of fetal development, could be enough to cause or contribute to a learning or developmental disorder.

Something else to consider is that most drugs—both prescription and over-the-counter—are not recommended for the pregnant and nursing mother, unless absolutely necessary. While all medications have some unwanted side effects, they also have some value and none are considered nearly as poisonous as mercury. Yet pro-amalgam dentists have no qualms about exposing women who are pregnant and nursing to toxic amounts of mercury during the placement and unsafe removal of amalgam fillings. I cannot find a logical explanation for this.

Testing the Mother and Baby

In Appendix A: "Testing for Mercury" I discuss the more commonly available tests for mercury. But it's important to introduce the subject here because some of the tests also prove that mercury is being eliminated from the body. Of course, if mercury is being eliminated, it means mercury has to already be there. It's known that if you have amalgam fillings, 80 percent of the mercury released from them enters your body. It's also known that if it's entering your body, the fetus and nursing baby will also be exposed to significant amounts of it.

In my opinion, the best test for this purpose is the fecal metals test, because it is a very safe and accurate way to determine if mercury is being removed from the mother and baby. It doesn't require a pharmaceutical chelator, making it an ideal test for a pregnant or nursing mother and a baby. As it's difficult to diagnose autism at a very early age, testing the baby for mercury using the non-invasive fecal metals test could serve as an early indicator of an increased risk for learning and developmental disorders.

The test can demonstrate whether high or low amounts of mercury are being eliminated. I say "low amounts" because studies show that many autistic children have much lower plasma levels of glutathione (GSH), and the substances needed to make GSH, than children without autism. Thus, the fecal metals test would be a useful indicator for determining if the baby is able to eliminate mercury. In fact, if the mother also took the fecal metals test, and she showed high amounts of mercury being released while the baby showed abnormally low levels, it could be an indication that the baby isn't able to remove mercury. Of course, this test would need to be evaluated by a qualified health professional, one who is also familiar with autism.

Another benefit of this test is that if you know your baby is eliminating mercury, it will allow you to initiate treatment to increase the baby's ability to remove it, possibly before the symptoms of autism or any learning or developmental disorder develop. You'll find some resources at the end of the chapter for gathering additional information about treating autism. One excellent study by Dr. Amy Holmes showed that if treatment for chronic mercury poisoning begins soon enough, many of the early symptoms attributed to autism can be reversed. More information about Dr. Holmes is found at the end of this chapter.

Early Signs and Symptoms of Autism

Generally, autism isn't diagnosed until about age three, but in addition to the fecal metals test, some early signs and symptoms can be useful indicators of autism.

- no smiling or joyful expressions by six months
- no babbling by 12 months
- no pointing or using other gestures by 12 months
- not using single words by 16 months
- not using two-word phrases by 24 months
- any loss of speech, language, or social skills at any age

Suggestions for Minimizing the Mother's Risk of Mercury Exposure

If you're planning a family, I can offer the following suggestions. First and foremost, have your mercury fillings safely removed and replaced as far in advance as possible prior to conception. Second, participate in a mercury detoxification program as soon as possible prior to becoming pregnant.

I realize that the preventive approach to removing a major source of mercury isn't possible for those who are now pregnant and those who are nursing their children. Over the years, many women who were pregnant or nursing have asked my advice about having their mercury fillings removed during this period. I've seen no evidence that pro-amalgam dentists are concerned about removing or putting in these fillings. But I do believe that the general consensus among mercury safe dentists is that a pregnant or nursing mother shouldn't have her amalgam fillings placed or removed during this period. This lack of consensus can create confusion, and while I can provide you with information that could help you understand this issue, the decision will be yours to make.

Utilizing a safe removal protocol to remove your amalgam fillings will reduce your exposure to mercury during their removal by up to 90 percent or more. The 10 percent you could receive would have to be weighed against the total amount of mercury you'd take in during the time the fillings were left in place. Based on the available information, an amalgam filling left in the mother's mouth for the entire period of fetal development and nursing would expose the mother, fetus, and nursing baby to a far greater amount of mercury than having that filling safely removed. But the safe removal protocol must be strictly followed. It is explained in detail in Chapter 8: "Safely Removing Mercury Amalgam (Silver) Fillings."

While the one-time exposure to mercury on the day of amalgam removal may be greater than the total amount the mother would receive from the filling on that particular day, removal would eliminate all future exposure the fetus and nursing baby would receive from it. Given mercury's poisonous effect on the fetus during this critically important developmental period, this is an important option to consider. However, if a number of fillings are to be removed, their removal should be spaced out over time, minimizing the larger exposure that could occur by removing too many fillings at one sitting. As the fillings are removed, the mother will be better able to deal with the mercury continuing to enter her body from the fillings still remaining. I cannot tell you what to do but I also suggest that you consult with your physician prior to making any decisions regarding removing your amalgam fillings during pregnancy and nursing.

If you decide *not* to have your fillings removed, I urge you to *strictly* follow the guidelines I've established to minimize the amount of mercury released from your fillings while they are still in your teeth (see Chapter 10: "Reducing Mercury Exposure from Amalgam (Silver) Fillings").

Remember that removing the fillings isn't the same as removing the accumulated mercury in your body. But because stored mercury is bound so tightly to where it's attached, it isn't that much of a threat to the fetus or nursing baby. Mercury that's attached to proteins or enzymes doesn't just jump off and roam through the body, and you can take some comfort in that fact.

By far the greatest threat to the fetus or nursing baby isn't from what's stored in the mother's body but what's released from her fillings and enters her body daily. It's the mercury that hasn't yet attached to a protein or enzyme in the mother that is the problem.

Summing It Up

In my opinion, the effects of chronic exposure to mercury during fetal development and nursing must be included as the primary cause of, or significant contributor to, autism and all other learning and developmental disorders. It's clear that for mothers with amalgam fillings, the major source of mercury exposure to the fetus and nursing baby will come from their fillings. Yet, in spite of the evidence, the ADA and its pro-amalgam supporters continue to say that the amount of mercury released from amalgam fillings isn't great enough to be considered a health hazard for anyone but those "few" who are allergic to it. I also thought you'd find it interesting that as recently as May 2005, the ADA endorsed amalgam as being safe for pregnant women.

We know that mercury is released from amalgam fillings and how toxic it is to the fetus and nursing baby. Although definitive scientific studies haven't yet been done to conclusively prove that mercury from amalgam fillings is the main cause of autism, I believe there is enough information available to support that conclusion.

That said, I want you to know that my intention here is not to criticize or judge any mother who had amalgam fillings while pregnant or nursing. You cannot assume responsibility for what you didn't know or couldn't control. *You are the victim here!* In my opinion, the blame rests squarely on dentists who've taken an oath to educate their patients about issues that can affect their patients' oral and overall health, and did not do so!

Resources

If you have an autistic child, it isn't enough to talk about the cause or its prevention. This is an issue I'm deeply concerned about, and while I'm not an expert in autism or its treatment, I've included some resources you may find helpful.

Dr. Amy Holmes. Her website deals brilliantly with the subject of chelating (removing) mercury from the autistic child. A physician and mother of an autistic child, Dr. Holmes has explored the testing and treatment for mercury poisoning in autistic spectrum children for many years. She is a world-renowned practitioner of oral chelation for children showing evidence of mercury poisoning. Dr. Holmes was also one of a group of noted physicians who pioneered a new direction in mercury detoxification of autistic children based on careful attention to testing and nutrient/mineral supplementation. You can read more about this at www.healing-arts.org/children/holmes.htm.

While Dr. Holmes no longer has an active practice, you can learn more about her and how to find other health practitioners involved with treating autism by visiting www.healing-arts.org/children/amyholmes.htm.

Talk About Curing Autism (TACA). This organization provides valuable information on improving the quality of life for people with autism. www.tacanow.com

The Healing Center Online. This site offers useful information about alternative therapies for treating children with developmental delays and other neurometabolic conditions and disorders. www.healing-arts.org/children/index.htm.

Relationship of Vaccinations to Autism. One of the best sources of information about all aspects of autism, especially its relationship to mercury from vaccinations. This excellent research paper compares the symptoms of autism to those of early chronic mercury poisoning and is provided by Sallie Bernard and other researchers and health professionals in this field. www.vaccinationnews.com/DailyNews/July2001/AutismUniqueMercPoison.htm.

SafeMinds (Sensible Action For Ending Mercury-Induced Neurological Disorders). This private nonprofit organization was founded by Sallie Bernard and others to investigate and raise awareness of the risks to infants and children of exposure to mercury from medical products, including thimerosal in vaccines. SafeMinds supports research on the potential harmful effects of mercury in thimerosal. www.safeminds.org.

Dr. Nicola McFadzean. This website discusses the various laboratory tests for autism, such as blood, urine, stool, saliva, and hair. www.drnicola.com/5901/14001.html.

Arizona State University's Autism/Asperger's Research Program. This website discusses the many treatment options for mercury/metal toxicity in autism and related developmental disorders. www.eas.asu.edu/~autism.

You'll find many more websites about autism than those listed here, but these are the ones I recommend starting with. And while they're not in any particular order, they are all very informative and useful. A word of caution, though—I recommend that you print any information you feel is important. Although these sites have been around for a number of years and are well regarded, websites do come and go.

What's Next

It's one thing to be made aware of a problem, and quite another to be offered a solution. So far I've dealt with the many health issues related to mercury exposure from amalgam fillings. By now you're well aware that these poisonous fillings shouldn't be in your garage, let alone your teeth. The next chapter will begin the solution process, starting with how to find a mercury free and mercury safe dentist.

Seven

Finding a Mercury Free and Mercury Safe Dentist

Hopefully you've decided to have your mercury amalgam fillings removed. Great! But you still have one more crucial step to go—finding a mercury free and mercury safe dentist. Having these fillings removed unsafely will expose you to extraordinarily high amounts of mercury, so it's vital to your health to find a dentist who removes amalgams in a safe way. And it will be a lot easier to find mercury safe dentists if you know what they do, how they do it, and why.

This chapter will explain the difference between pro-amalgam and mercury free/mercury safe dentists. It will also inform you how you can deal with obstacles to safely removing and replacing amalgam fillings with safe alternatives. A mercury safe dentist is one who is aware of the health hazards of mercury vapor, doesn't use amalgam in his or her practice, and knows how to minimize your exposure to mercury vapor by safely removing these toxic fillings. Chapter 8: "Safely Removing Amalgam (Silver) Fillings" discusses the safe removal protocol in detail.

When all is said and done, removing and replacing your amalgam fillings doesn't have anything to do with whether they are in good shape from a structural standpoint. Safely removing amalgam fillings isn't about the health of the filling, but about protecting you from excessive exposure to mercury during their removal.

Mercury Free and Mercury Safe: What's in a Name?

Strictly speaking, the term "mercury free" refers to dentists who don't put amalgam fillings in their patients' teeth. But over time, the term came to encompass those who not only didn't put them into their patients teeth, but those who also safely removed them.

However, mercury free isn't really an accurate description, because as long as dentists still remove amalgam fillings, their offices can't officially be called "mercury free." Therefore, *mercury safe* is a more accurate description of those who not only don't put them in, but also remove them as safely as possible. Thus I use the term "mercury safe" throughout the book to describe a dentist who doesn't use amalgam and safely removes these fillings.

Today it's even more important to know the difference between a mercury free and mercury safe dentist. More and more dentists are no longer using amalgam, because it simply isn't a good filling when compared to the newer composites. Increasingly, these dentists refer to their practices as being mercury free. However, that doesn't mean that they believe mercury fillings are a health hazard, or that they will protect you from excessive exposure to mercury during their removal. Bottom line . . . you can't assume that a dentist who advertises his or her practice as being mercury *free* is also mercury *safe*.

The Importance of Safely Removing Mercury Fillings

Being protected during the amalgam removal process is *extremely* important, because the greatest exposure to mercury vapor occurs when these fillings are removed. When a mercury safe dentist uses a safe amalgam removal protocol, the amount of mercury vapor you would be exposed to can be reduced by up to 90 percent or more. The importance of this protection can be better understood when you realize that unsafely drilling out an amalgam filling can release up to 4,000 mcg of mercury vapor. As you read in Chapter 2, that's an enormous amount of mercury. Dentists who are committed to mercury safe dentistry are concerned about protecting not only their patients from mercury exposure, but also themselves, their staff, and the environment.

All three are obviously important considerations, but your primary concern is to make sure *you* are being protected. As long as a dentist is doing his or her best to minimize *your* mercury exposure, you can't ask for more than that. Minimizing exposure to mercury vapor during removal is important to everyone, but even more so for pregnant women, nursing mothers, those whose immune systems are compromised, and especially those who are allergic to mercury.

To date, none of the dental schools, the American Dental Association (ADA), or any government regulatory agency have established, or even suggested, a protocol for safely removing amalgam fillings. Thus, no dentist is legally required to offer patients any protection against mercury exposure when removing their amalgam fillings.

The Difference between a Mercury Safe and a Pro-Amalgam Dentist

By the third year of dental school, every dental student knows how to remove and replace amalgam fillings. Every pro-amalgam dentist removes and replaces old amalgam fillings with new amalgams many times a day. Removing amalgams without using a safe protocol is a simple and quick process. But what really separates mercury safe and pro-amalgam dentists is that mercury safe dentists know that:

- amalgam fillings are a health hazard

- the mercury released from amalgam fillings negatively affects your health

- you need to be protected from exposure to mercury vapor during the removal process

Mercury safe dentists also have the specialized equipment, training, experience, and skills necessary to protect you from excessive exposure to mercury during amalgam removal.

While I absolutely respect the right of pro-amalgam dentists to expose themselves to mercury, I don't believe they have the right to expose their patients, their staff, and the environment to mercury—just because they choose to believe what the ADA tells them regarding the safety of amalgam fillings.

It's one thing to believe that the mercury released from a patient's amalgam fillings on a daily basis isn't a health hazard. But it's another thing entirely not to offer the patient protection against mercury exposure during the removal process. These are two separate issues because there's a *huge* difference between the amount of mercury emitted from the fillings on a daily basis and the amount released during their removal at the dental office.

I can't stress enough the importance of finding a mercury safe dentist who has the qualifications to safely remove your amalgam fillings. It may cost a little more to get this kind of protection, but it's well worth it. Another advantage of going to a mercury safe dentist is that you won't have to debate why you believe amalgam fillings are a health hazard, why you want them removed, and why you want to minimize your exposure to mercury in the process. In fact, no regulatory agency, scientist, or health professional would ever suggest not doing everything possible to minimize your exposure to mercury, except for one group—pro-amalgam dentists.

A Mercury Safe Dentist by Other Names

Mercury safe dentists may also refer to themselves by other names. Some of the more common ones are: holistic, biological, alternative, natural, and metal free. To date, there are no universally accepted definitions for these terms, or standards that must be adhered to. Thus, the distinctions aren't always clear. But regardless of whatever other term is used, I consider all mercury safe dentists to be "holistic" dentists, and refer to them as such.

The following is a partial list of therapies that a mercury safe dentist may offer in addition to a safe removal protocol, and I believe that the dentist of the future will offer many, if not all, of the therapies listed below. Thankfully there are holistic and biological dentists who are providing these services today. (These therapies are meant to support dental treatment and aren't considered substitutes for it.) Regardless of the additional services a mercury safe dentist offers, the most important benefit is the safe removal of your amalgam fillings. (Even today, some dentists have studied some, or all, of these therapies.)

Alternative Dental Therapies	
Acupuncture	Electro-Dermal Screening
Applied Kinesiology	Homeopathy
Biocompatibility Testing	Mercury Detoxification
Cavitation Diagnosis	Metal-Free Restorations
Cranial Sacral Therapy	Neuro Muscular Therapy

How to Find a Mercury Safe Dentist

As of 2008, 52 percent of practicing general dentists in the United States no longer use amalgam and can rightfully call themselves mercury free. But based on my research, only about 15 percent of them are currently mercury *safe*. This number is on the rise, but it still means that it isn't always easy to find a mercury safe dentist, especially in smaller towns and rural areas. But with a little effort, it's not impossible to find one in your area.

To help your search, I founded the International Association of Mercury Free Dentists (IAMFD), an association listing mercury free/mercury safe dentists worldwide. The directory is one of the largest worldwide listings of mercury safe dentists and you can access the list of members at www.dentalwellness4u.com. All members have an expanded listing which includes information about them, their services, and a link to their websites, if applicable. This extensive information will help you evaluate what they offer prior to contacting them, and no other mercury free listing service provides such detailed information.

While the listing on my website is extensive, it doesn't yet account for all the mercury safe dentists. If you can't find a mercury safe dentist listed in your city, don't despair. I suggest that you first check my website for the dentist closest to your city or town. Second, call that mercury safe office, tell the receptionist where you found out about them, and then ask to be referred to a mercury safe dentist closer to your immediate area. Mercury safe dentists are a great referral source for each other.

Another great way to find a mercury safe dentist is by word of mouth. Check with your friends, fellow employees, and family members to see if they know of a dentist who is mercury safe. But if you still can't find a mercury safe dentist near you, it would be worth it, if at all possible, to travel to the closest one you can find.

Overcoming the Obstacles

For many people, finding a mercury safe dentist is just the first hurdle to jump in having their amalgam fillings safely removed. For some there's the cost factor. For others it may be fear of going to the dentist. And then there are those who feel it makes more financial sense to wait until their amalgam fillings wear out before replacing them. So let's look at these barriers and see what can be done to overcome them.

Now or Later

The most important factor to consider is that the sooner you have your amalgam fillings removed, the less mercury you will be exposed to. It's *always* best to quickly and safely remove the source of exposure to any toxic substance. The more toxic the substance, the greater the need to remove it as quickly as possible. The longer you wait, the more detrimental it will be to your health. In this case, what might be okay for your teeth is definitely not okay for your body!

Dental Costs vs. Health Care Costs

If you fully understand the health issues involved and have already committed to having your mercury fillings removed, I don't think cost needs to get in the way. Mercury filling removal isn't elective or cosmetic dentistry—it's mandatory for health. This isn't a matter of paying to have your fillings replaced so you can look better and have movie-star teeth. Regardless of how much it costs, I believe the concern for your immediate and long-term health will help motivate you to have these poisonous fillings replaced with a safe alternative.

There's another argument for not waiting to have your fillings removed: Mercury fillings aren't permanent. Their average life expectancy is about 8 to 12 years, though I've seen some that need replacing much sooner and others lasting much longer. Depending on their age, chances are you'll need to have your amalgam fillings removed and replaced at some point. So the real question is when.

The question of cost actually needs to be reframed. When you compare the cost of replacing these toxic fillings against the long-term cost of treating health issues related to chronic mercury poisoning, the picture looks quite different. There's no doubt the long-term cost of health care far exceeds that of dental treatment. Consider, for example, the long-term treatment cost for any of the symptoms and diseases related to chronic mercury poisoning—such as chronic fatigue syndrome, heart disease, multiple sclerosis, or autism.

Another consideration is quality of life. If you're now dealing with any symptoms or diseases directly or indirectly related to chronic mercury poisoning, removing your amalgam fillings will improve the quality of your life. How can you put a price tag on that? So when you think of having your mercury fillings removed, think *quality of life*. And don't forget to include prevention in this process, because preventing a health problem from happening will *always* end up costing less than treatment. It really is true that an ounce of prevention is worth a pound of cure!

What It Will Cost

The dental filling most commonly used to replace an amalgam filling is called a composite. Generally, the apples-to-apples cost of using a composite to replace an amalgam can range from 25 to 100 percent more. If the amalgam being replaced is too large to be functionally restored with a composite, the filling of choice would be a gold onlay, gold crown, porcelain to metal crown, or a metal-free crown, inlay, or onlay. Crowns and onlays are considerably more expensive than composites, and their cost will vary depending on where you live. You'll find my recommendations for replacing mercury amalgam fillings in Chapter 9: "Replacing Your Amalgam (Silver) Fillings."

One of the most commonly asked cost questions is why mercury safe dentists charge more than pro-amalgam dentists. The answer is straightforward:

- Mercury safe dentists invest more in education and specialized equipment that allows them to safely remove the fillings

- It takes more time to safely remove amalgams

- The materials used in composites are more expensive than those used in amalgams

Practically speaking, the additional material and equipment costs, and the investment these dentists must make in education, mean that they are more experienced and better equipped to safely remove and replace amalgam fillings with safe ones. But remember, pro-amalgam dentists also charge more for replacing an amalgam with a composite, but don't provide a safe removal protocol.

How to Pay for It

If the cost of removing amalgam fillings is still prohibitive, you do have other options to consider. First, discuss your financial situation with your dentist. Ask if he or she is open to a monthly payment plan. This way you could have all your mercury fillings removed in the shortest period of time but spread the cost out over a longer period of time. Some dental offices are agreeable to this and some aren't, but it's worth discussing. Dentists will generally be more open to this form of payment if it doesn't involve the costly laboratory expenses related to producing cast inlays, onlays, crowns, and bridges. If it does, the dentist may still work with you but may ask that you pay for the laboratory costs up front. Nothing is etched in stone and many dental offices are willing to negotiate.

For some people, removing these toxic fillings is so important that they're willing to borrow money in order to have it done as quickly as possible. This is especially true for those who have any of the more obvious symptoms or diseases related to chronic mercury poisoning. The drawback that borrowing entails is the interest rate you may be required to pay—but that has to be weighed against long-term health issues and their related costs.

If you're reasonably healthy and you haven't reached the point where you're experiencing many mercury related symptoms, you could spread out the cost by spacing the removal out over time. But remember, you are still being poisoned by the fillings that remain in your teeth.

Dental Insurance Companies

I'm often asked if dental insurance will pay for the removal of mercury fillings and their replacements with safe ones. Although they don't answer to the ADA, the majority of dental insurance companies basically take the same approach—they consider mercury fillings to be a safe and inexpensive filling (with the emphasis here on "inexpensive"). Thus, they say there is no reason to pay for amalgam removal and replacement with more costly fillings solely because of health concerns. It doesn't matter to a dental insurance company that you test positive for mercury poisoning or have symptoms of chronic mercury poisoning. After all, replacing amalgams with a safe filling material will be more costly for the insurance company.

In the future the situation could change, so it doesn't hurt to ask your dental insurance company. But don't get your hopes up. The sad reality is that dental insurance companies exist to make a profit, not to improve your health. However, when mercury fillings are finally banned, insurance companies will have no choice but to pay for their replacement.

While dental insurance companies won't pay for amalgam removal for health reasons, they are obligated to pay for replacement of worn out, fractured, or broken amalgams. The chances of this happening are greatest for fillings more than eight years old. The best thing to do is to specifically ask your mercury safe dentist to evaluate your fillings for wear and other structural problems. If the insurance company accepts the dentist's findings that your amalgam fillings need to be replaced because of structural problems or because they've worn out, it will have to pay for replacing them. However, most companies will only pay for the cost of a new amalgam, so be prepared to pay for the difference between the cost of an amalgam and the cost of a composite.

Health Insurance Companies

Dental insurance companies may never see the financial benefit in replacing amalgam fillings for health reasons. But that doesn't mean *health* insurance companies won't soon get the message. Once these companies realize they're collectively paying billions of dollars a year for health care costs related to chronic mercury poisoning, I think they'll gladly help cover, or share, the removal cost. After all, it's your *body* that's being poisoned by mercury, not your teeth.

It's my hope that health insurance companies will ultimately see amalgam filling removal as a necessary medical procedure, one essential to preventing chronic mercury poisoning and its many related health problems. But don't hold your breath. I still haven't discovered why, but many health insurance companies haven't embraced the concept of paying a little to prevent what otherwise will end up costing them a lot. Even so, there are signs that their attitude regarding prevention is changing.

Businesses that self-fund their dental and health plans aren't at the mercy of dental insurance companies and can be more flexible. When a self-funded company initiates a dental wellness program—one designed to educate employees about the health benefits of safely removing amalgam fillings and preventing gum disease—the company could not only save up to 60 percent on dental care costs, but also reduce health care costs directly related to dental disease by at least 20 percent. The benefit of doing so is that the considerable savings in this area will be retained as profit.

I've developed an employee education program that is the most practical and cost-effective way to reduce dental and related health care costs. If you are employed by a company whose dental plan is self-funded and want to learn how to significantly lower your company's dental and health care costs, please call me at 800-335-7755.

Dealing with Fear and Anxiety

While I don't know with certainty, estimates say that up to 50 percent of the U.S. population has some fear or anxiety about going to the dentist. I'm one of those whose fear of dental treatment kept me from going to the dentist for many years, and I personally think the percentage is higher. Regardless of a few percentage points here and there, over 100 million people in the U.S. could delay or avoid necessary dental treatment because of fear. Any number of fears—pain, injections, drills, noise, the cost, or even confinement in the dental chair—can keep someone from seeking necessary dental treatment.

It's bad enough to put off needed treatment for tooth decay and gum disease, but it will be far more disastrous if a dental fear or phobia prevents you from having your mercury fillings safely removed and replaced. Whatever your particular fear, it can be dealt with, at least to the degree that it doesn't stop you from having these poison-laced fillings removed from your teeth.

One of the most important steps you can take for dealing with any dental fear you have is to talk to your dentist. Your dentist can help you, but only if he or she knows about your concerns. It isn't silly or cowardly to admit it, and you needn't be embarrassed. What you absolutely should never do is let it get in the way of improving your health and extending your life expectancy. (See Appendix C for more information about the relationship of oral health to overall health.)

When you go for your first appointment, tell your dentist what your fears are before you begin treatment. You'll be amazed at how he or she—using modern, stress-free, pain-free, high-tech dentistry—can help you overcome your fears. If you're dealing with fear and your dentist isn't willing to work with you, I recommend finding one who is.

What's Next

The next chapter deals with the safe protocol for removing mercury fillings. There's more to removing mercury fillings than just drilling them out, and you should know what can be done to protect you.

Eight

Safely Removing Mercury Amalgam (Silver) Fillings

I've spoken with thousands of people over the past 30 years and discovered that the majority of them don't realize that amalgam fillings are harmful to their health. Most don't even know that 50 percent of their amalgam (silver) filling is mercury. Still more people don't know that amalgams give off toxic mercury vapor, and the fraction who do know don't realize how much vapor these fillings release when removed without a safe protocol.

For example, the World Health Organization (WHO) estimates that those with amalgam fillings receive up to 17 mcg of mercury per day from their fillings. *That pales in comparison to the 4,000 mcg of mercury released when an amalgam filling is unsafely removed.* The good news here is that when a dentist uses a safe removal protocol it can reduce your exposure to mercury vapor during the removal process by up to 90 percent or more. So, given the vast amount of mercury that can be released during amalgam removal, it's imperative to understand the difference between the safe removal procedures that mercury safe dentists use and what pro-amalgam dentists do (or rather, don't do).

To date, the mercury safe dental community hasn't reached a universal consensus on a protocol for minimizing a patient's exposure to mercury during amalgam removal. But the International Academy of Oral Medicine and Toxicology (IAOMT), a network of dental, medical, and research professionals, has established what I believe to be the best guidelines for safely removing these fillings. My research has shown that their guidelines are those most often incorporated by mercury safe dentists when developing their own removal protocols.

The guidelines I recommend for safe amalgam filling removal have been taken from several sources: the IAOMT, my own experience and research, and other prominent holistic and biological dental organizations. While using this preventive approach to minimizing mercury vapor exposure is important for everyone, it's an absolute must for those who:

- are pregnant or nursing

- suspect or know they are allergic to mercury

- have ever had any adverse side effects during or after having amalgam fillings placed or removed

- have a compromised immune system, numerous allergies, or other serious health problems

Some dentists don't follow every one of the guidelines I list in the following section, while others go even further. I believe the IAOMT protocol is more than adequate and should be acceptable to most dentists who subscribe to the basic concepts of mercury safe dentistry.

Still, new information emerges each year about the safest way to remove amalgam fillings, and it's possible that a new technique or approach may be added after the publication of this book. Thus, if your dentist says he or she is mercury safe but deviates from the protocol I've included, it doesn't mean his or her protocol won't be effective. But if it varies too much, make sure you get a satisfactory explanation as to why.

Mercury Amalgam Fillings: Safe Removal Protocol

There are 11 procedures that most mercury safe dentists use to minimize mercury exposure to the patient, the dental staff, and the environment during amalgam filling removal. They are divided into four categories:

- minimizing the amount of mercury that could be released from the filling

- intercepting the mercury that escapes the filling before the patient breathes it in

- filtering the office air

• cleaning the patient and disposing of contaminated material, such as patient coverings, gloves, and rubber dam

1. Cooling the Fillings

The amount of mercury vapor released from an amalgam filling is directly proportionate to its temperature. Drilling out an amalgam filling generates a *tremendous* amount of heat. Cooling the filling by using as much water as possible during the process will significantly reduce the amount of mercury vapor released.

2. Chunking Amalgams

Mercury safe dentists use a removal process called "chunking" in which they use a special drill bit to section the filling into large chunks. These chunks can then be easily removed by a hand instrument or suction, which reduces drilling time and therefore the amount of mercury vapor released.

3. Using High-Volume Evacuation

Mercury safe dentists use a powerful suction/vacuum system. This important piece of equipment minimizes your exposure to mercury vapor because in effect it intercepts the vapor before you can breathe it in. The tip of the suction/vacuum hose will be placed as close to the filling as possible during the entire removal process. This procedure captures most of the mercury vapor and particles released as the filling is removed.

4. Providing an Alternative Source of Air

All mercury safe dentists adhere to the first three protocols, but not always this fourth one—giving you an alternative source of air to breathe. Some feel that as long as the first three procedures are strictly followed, this isn't necessary. But if any one of the first three procedures isn't followed, you should request an alternative source of air during the *entire* removal process. If your mercury safe dentist doesn't provide one, be sure to ask him or her if they're using a high-volume evacuation system and if the other protective methods listed above are being used. However, if you are in the high risk category, especially if you are pregnant or nursing, I would insist on an alternative source of air.

An alternative source of air is provided by a nasal hood, which covers your nose. Through this hood you breathe either compressed air or oxygen from a tank. I don't believe an alternative source of air is necessary after the fillings have been removed.

You should always concentrate on breathing through your nostrils and *avoid breathing through your mouth* while your mercury fillings are being removed—whether you are provided with an alternative source of air or not.

5. Using a Rubber Dam

The rubber dam was designed to isolate the tooth or teeth being worked on, making it easier for the dentist to see and protect the tooth/teeth from bacteria, moisture, and the tongue. The rubber dam is made from either latex rubber or silicone for those allergic to latex. It is very thin and flexible, comes in various colors, and can range in size from 5 x 5 inch to 6 x 6 inch squares. Until recently, dentists believed that the rubber dam would protect the patient from inhaling mercury vapor through the mouth. It's now known that mercury vapor can readily pass through a rubber dam made from latex, the most common rubber dam material. (Silicone is more resistant to mercury vapor.)

A large percentage of patients believe that the rubber dam offers the greatest protection from mercury vapor and insist that it be used. But because the rubber dam doesn't actually protect you from inhaling mercury vapor, it isn't absolutely necessary for the safe removal of amalgam fillings. Although the rubber dam offers little protection against mercury vapor, it does make it easier to evacuate the filling material and prevent amalgam particles from being swallowed. Amalgam particles can't be absorbed into the body, but it's always wise to avoid swallowing any dental material.

More and more dentists are now using a dental device called the Isolite System that illuminates and isolates the tooth and provides a constant source of suction close to the amalgam. It's often used in place of the rubber dam, and I believe it's more effective at protecting the patient from mercury vapor and amalgam particles. As a rule of thumb, when it comes to choosing between the rubber dam and any alternative, I recommend trusting your mercury safe dentist to decide when and which one is or isn't necessary—but if in doubt, ask for an explanation.

6. Cleaning Up Immediately

Once the removal process is completed, the dentist and assistant should remove and dispose of their gloves and the rubber dam (if used) and thoroughly rinse and vacuum your entire mouth for at least 10 seconds. This process helps remove amalgam particles and residual mercury captured by the saliva. You should make every effort not to swallow during the short rinsing procedure. When this is finished, take a *small* amount of water and gargle as far back into your throat as possible. Once you've gargled, don't swallow this watery residue! It should be evacuated by the dental assistant, or spit into a cup.

In addition, when the removal procedure is finished, the dentist or dental assistant should remove and dispose of your protective covering and clean your face and neck. All mercury safe dentists should routinely do this, but remind the assistant if she or he forgets. After all, you don't want to take any mercury home with you.

7. Using Additional Air Purification
Some mercury safe dentists use an additional air filtering system that's placed as close to the patient's mouth as is practical. The more popular ones resemble an elephant's trunk and have an opening about 4 inches in diameter. This filter is helpful, but there are other mercury safe dentists who believe that the patient can be adequately protected without such a system. More and more mercury safe dentists are using this type of office purification system, and while it's a positive addition to the basic removal protocol, I believe this system is more effective at protecting the dentist and assistant than the patient.

8. Filtering Air in the Dental Operatory
Many mercury safe dental offices filter the office air because they work in it all day and it's to their benefit to do so. Thus, doing this is more important for the dentist and staff than it is for you. Although mercury safe offices don't put in amalgam fillings, they certainly remove them. You should be encouraged by the fact that mercury safe dentists also want to take the necessary precautions to protect themselves and their entire staff from excessive exposure to mercury.

9. Using Activated Charcoal
Although definitive studies haven't been done, there is some evidence that shows that activated charcoal taken 10–15 minutes before amalgam removal can capture swallowed elemental mercury and mercury vapor, allowing it to be harmlessly passed out of the intestine via the feces. I consider this to be optional, as only 0.01 percent of swallowed elemental mercury is absorbed through the intestine. But it can't hurt to add it, especially if you are in the high mercury risk category.

10. Vitamin C Infusions
Some dentists and health professionals consider vitamin C (ascorbic acid) infusions to be an effective method of protecting the body from mercury vapor during the process of removing amalgam fillings. Based on my evaluation of

the available data, those who support the vitamin C protocol believe that it can protect the body from mercury vapor when it is in the bloodstream. While I don't consider this an essential procedure for the majority of patients, if you're allergic to mercury, have numerous symptoms and diseases related to chronic mercury poisoning, or have a compromised immune system, I would recommend these infusions, if available.

Since it's administered intravenously, a vitamin C infusion needs to be coordinated with your dentist and a qualified health practitioner. To date, few dental offices offer this service. But if you feel vitamin C protection would be beneficial and can't find a dentist who will arrange an infusion, you can take an oral dose. However, this method is less effective because the blood levels of vitamin C obtained with an infusion would be significantly higher than from an oral dose. Still, oral vitamin C could provide some additional protection from mercury vapor while it's in the bloodstream.

Before doing this, discuss it with your dentist. If you are in agreement, obtain a packet of powdered vitamin C from a health food store and take it with you to the dental office. After the area to be treated has been effectively numbed, dissolve the powdered vitamin C in a glass of water and drink it as soon as possible before the removal procedure begins. Because vitamin C may diminish the effect of the anesthetic in some people, I recommend taking it after the anesthetic has been given and the part of you mouth being worked on is numbed. This method works better on an empty stomach because vitamin C is quickly absorbed from the intestine into the blood stream if no other food is present in the stomach.

11. Supplements

I recommend that everyone start a mercury detoxification program before the fillings are removed. I suggest that you at least take the supplements listed in Chapter 11, page 117, as many days prior to amalgam removal as possible, except for vitamin C on the day of your appointment for amalgam removal.

Comments from Dr. Tom

Remember, no dentist, even those who are mercury safe, is under any legal obligation to provide patients with protection against mercury exposure during the removal process. Mercury safe dentists provide this service because they believe mercury is a powerful poison and feel they have a moral obligation to minimize their patients' exposure to it.

As for the safe removal protocols I've discussed, what I've presented are only suggested guidelines—and there may be variations on these I've listed that are equally effective. It should also be noted that these procedures are not all weighted equally in regard to the degree of protection from mercury vapor and particles provided. For example, it's much more important for the dentist to chunk out the fillings than for you to take activated charcoal. It's also more beneficial to you if your dentist keeps the fillings cool and uses a high-speed evacuator and alternative source of air than if he or she filters the dental office air.

From a patient's perspective, not all these procedures may be absolutely necessary to safely remove amalgam fillings, but the more of them your mercury safe dentist uses, the better for everyone. And remember, if you're unsure about *any* procedure your mercury safe dentist is using, ask for an explanation.

What to Watch Out For

If asked, some dentists who don't use mercury but are not mercury safe will abide by your decision to remove your amalgam fillings because of your health concerns. But it's unlikely they will have the equipment and experience needed to remove them safely. Also, pro-amalgam dentists don't believe these fillings are a health hazard and don't understand the importance of following a safe removal procedure or protecting you. If your present dentist falls into one of these categories, then my first recommendation is that you find another one who is well versed in a safe removal protocol. After all, it's your body, you hire the dentist, and it's *your* decision to make.

If circumstances dictate that you absolutely must work with a dentist who isn't mercury safe, even though he or she is mercury free, you can provide a copy of the safe removal guidelines presented here and ask that he or she follow them as closely as possible.

For Mercury Free Dentists and Patients

If you're looking for a mercury safe dentist, you'll find an extensive listing on my website, www.dentalwellness4u.com. If you're a mercury safe dentist and want to join the ever-expanding mercury free and mercury safe dental community by becoming a member of the Mercury Free Dentist Internet Listing Service, please call me call toll free, 800-335-7755. I also recommend that you visit my website to learn more about the benefits of membership.

What's Next?

Now that you know how to find mercury safe dentists and the steps they take to safely remove amalgam fillings, the next logical step in the process is to learn about the fillings used to replace them.

Nine

Replacing Your Mercury Amalgam (Silver) Fillings

You've decided to have your amalgam fillings safely removed, you know what needs to be done to protect you from mercury vapor during their removal, and are now wondering what they should be replaced with. After all, refilling your teeth is just as important as "unfilling" them. Your mercury safe dentist will be able to offer the best refilling choices, and since mercury safe dentists don't place amalgam fillings, they're more likely to stay current on the latest in replacement filling materials.

While your mercury safe dentist will be the best source of information about replacing amalgams and will give you the best possible options (treatment plans), I think it will be useful for you to know a little about your choices. This information will help you work with your dentist to select the restoration that's right for you. But remember, I'm not your dentist and books don't have eyes, ears, or a mouth. The book can't look inside your mouth, and if your mercury safe dentist suggests a filling that doesn't match what I've discussed, I suggest you defer to him or her. If you are uncertain, ask that he or she explain the reasoning to you. Always remember that regardless of what type of restoration you choose to replace an amalgam filling, be sure to remind your dentist to always remove any remaining amalgam—and never, ever, ever, place any metal crown, or onlay, over an amalgam filling.

Composite Fillings

The composite filling is the material used most often to replace amalgams. Of course, you'll always find there are exceptions. For example, the composite should only be used if there's still enough tooth structure left to support the filling, and if there isn't, an onlay or crown is the best choice. I'll start with composites because they're so widely used and questions about their safety have recently been raised by some dentists and researchers.

Composites have truly revolutionized modern dentistry. Composite material has been available since the late 1950s and, due to the ever-increasing demand for it, it's constantly being improved. The latest generation of composites are far superior in regard to strength, durability, and adhesion to the tooth surface, than those used just 5 years ago. They're not only a vast improvement on earlier ones, but are also a far better filling material than mercury fillings in terms of function, aesthetics, and most importantly . . . safety.

Another important quality of composites is that preparing a tooth for a composite filling is far less invasive than preparing it for an amalgam filling, and significantly less tooth structure is lost in the process. A composite is also easy to repair if a piece chips off. Unlike amalgams, which don't bond to the tooth, the more recent generations of composites will strongly bond with the tooth structure, literally gluing the walls of the tooth and filling together, making the tooth a lot stronger than one with a comparable mercury filling.

However, placing a composite takes more skill, experience, and time than putting in a mercury filling, plus special equipment is needed. The additional time involved is due to the fact that a composite has to be placed in layers, and each layer has to be cured by a special light to harden it. As a result, the cost of a composite can be 25 to 100 percent more than a comparable amalgam. The lifespan of a composite varies from about 7 to 12 years—similar to an amalgam—and generally speaking, the smaller the composite, the longer it will last. But, most importantly, *composites don't release mercury vapor.*

Direct composites are placed in one appointment and will shrink slightly during the curing process and, unless properly placed, the integrity of the margin (where the filling meets the tooth) can be compromised. (I'll discuss the difference between "direct" and "indirect" composites later in this chapter.) Like any dental filling, composites need to be well cared for to prevent redecay. So if you are decay prone, you'll have to make sure you've established a good dental hygiene program.

Any filling material placed in, or over, a tooth can cause it to be sensitive to heat and cold, and composites are no exception. Sensitivity usually doesn't last more than 7 to 10 days but can last for up to 6 weeks. The key here is that the newly filled tooth should get progressively less sensitive each day. If the sensitivity doesn't decrease over time, or intensifies, make sure you immediately bring it to the attention of your dentist. Sensitivity is more likely to be experienced with fillings that are large, deep, and placed close to the nerve-rich dental pulp. If you've been sensitive to the placement of any dental restoration in the past, be sure to let your dentist know ahead of time, as there are ways to minimize sensitivity. Most dentists do this routinely, but it can't hurt to remind yours.

Composition of Composites

Composites consist of monomers (also referred to as a matrix or a binder) and fillers. In addition to monomers and fillers, composites also contain initiators and stabilizers. Initiators are light sensitive substances that promote the polymerization of the composite when cured with a light source, and stabilizers provide strength to the composite resin. Polymerization is a process where the same monomer is layered together many times to form a larger structure of the same material. Calcium carbonate, also know as limestone, is an example of a stabilizer.

The most common fillers are a combination of quartz, zinc glasses, lithium aluminum silicate, barium, and strontium. The most commonly used monomer is Bis-GMA, a compound composed of Bisphenol A (BPA) and glycidyl ester methacrylate (GMA). The chemical name for Bis-GMA is bisphenol A diglycidylether methacrylate. (Bisphenol A is an industrial chemical used primarily to make polycarbonate plastic and epoxy resins, including food packaging containers, plastic bottles, plastic toys, and water pipes.) In addition to Bis-GMA, you'll find a few other monomers used in composites—the Bisphenol dimethacrylates (Bis-DMA), ethylene glycol dimethacrylate (EGDMA), and triethylene glycol dimethacrylate (TEGDMA). When these materials are mixed together they form a paste-like substance. The paste is then applied to the tooth's cavity in layers. Each layer is then hardened, or "cured," by using an ultraviolet (UV) light, or a visible light source.

I know that these terms are quite a mouthful and I'll make every effort to simplify. Although I feel it will be helpful to those who want to do their own research on composite fillings, I fully understand if you decide to skip through this section and decide take the advice of your mercury safe dentist.

Health Effects of Bisphenol A (BPA)

In high concentrations, pure BPA can mimic the effects of estrogen. BPA is also known to be an endocrine disruptor, a term describing environmental chemicals that affect the endocrine system, such as the glands and hormones. Continuous exposure to high levels of BPA has also been associated with an increased risk of breast cancer. While we know that high levels of BPA can contribute to a number of health issues, there are questions about the impact of very low dosages of it. The most recent studies indicate that when it's combined with GMA, BPA isn't released as a vapor.

The Difference between Bis-GMA and Bisphenol A (BPA)

Bisphenol A is a component of Bis-GMA and not an isolated ingredient in composites. While more studies regarding this need to be done, we know:

- Manufacturers of composite material say there is no free, or un-reacted, BPA in the Bis-GMA or Bis-DMA monomers. This means that BPA is strongly bonded to another substance.

- Before BPA vapor can be released from a cured composite it would have to be heated to over 200° F/93° C.

- It would take a much stronger acid than is found in the stomach to dissolve swallowed composite particles and release free BPA.

- The amount of BPA detected from dental composites is 100 to 1,000 times lower than the level believed to be toxic.

Studies have shown that the Bis-GMA monomer in composites doesn't break down into its component parts and thus doesn't release BPA. A related factor to consider is whether or not the BPA that may be released from composites actually enters the body. One study showed that while low levels of BPA were detected in the saliva immediately after a composite was placed, no BPA was detected in the blood. This suggests that even if small amounts of BPA are released during placement of the composite, it doesn't access the blood stream and thus can't be considered a health hazard.

There are a number of studies supporting both the pro-BPA and anti-BPA positions, but from my analysis of the available research, there's nothing to support the concern that the small amount of BPA released from a composite filling is high enough to cause a health problem in the majority of the population. At this point, research indicates that the only time a person could possibly be exposed to BPA vapor from a composite is during the placement process. Studies show that some vapor is emitted from the composite until it is completely cured and hardened. The curing process for the latest versions of composites doesn't last long—a matter of seconds for smaller composites—so exposure to any free BPA during that period would be minimal.

If you're concerned about the possibility of BPA vapor exposure during the placement of a composite, I recommend asking your mercury safe dentist to use the same protection protocol for composites that he or she uses when removing mercury fillings—specifically providing an alternative source of air. Using an alternative source of air during placement of a composite can eliminate or minimize your exposure to BPA vapors. If you're pregnant or nursing, have numerous allergies, or a compromised immune system, you should request this extra protection.

Still Concerned?

If you're still concerned, you do have alternatives to BPA-based composites. Some composite materials on the market don't contain monomers of BPA. That doesn't mean that they're 100 percent safe for everyone, but at least it removes BPA from the equation. As of the publication of this book, two BPA-free direct composites are available: Diamondlite by Biodent, and Conquest Crystal (which has no metal products or Bis-GMA) by Jeneric Pentron Corporation.

At this time I currently know of one indirect composite material that doesn't contain Bis-GMA or other Bisphenol monomers—Sinfony by 3M ESPE. New composite materials are continually being developed, and if you have any question about whether this category of dental filling material is right for you, check with your mercury safe dentist.

Replacement Materials

While composites are the most common filling material used to replace mercury amalgam fillings, dentists also use ceramic, gold, and porcelain restorations. As always, if you have any questions about them, ask your mercury safe dentist to explain the advantages and disadvantages of any filling material he or she recommends.

Direct and Indirect Composites

Direct

Direct composites are placed in one appointment and are ideally suited for smaller fillings. Because they only involve one visit and have no associated laboratory costs, they are less expensive than an indirect composite. But they do have some drawbacks. Direct composites are technique sensitive, require more skill to place, and may not be as strong, or seal the border it forms with the tooth as effectively as an indirect composite.

Indirect

Indirect composites take two appointments to complete. They are used for larger cavities where an onlay or crown isn't required, but can also be used for smaller fillings. Preparing the tooth for an indirect composite is similar to preparing it for onlays or crown restorations.

With an indirect composite, the tooth is prepared, an impression is taken and sent to a dental laboratory. The finished composite is cemented into place just as a dental crown or cap would be. Indirect composites are made from either a composite or ceramic material. They are harder, stronger, and can last longer than a comparably sized direct composite. Most do not contain Bis-GMA or BPA, and if they do, they won't release BPA as a vapor because they are cured in a laboratory. In addition, the risk of sensitivity is minimized.

CEREC Restorations

CEREC is the acronym for a pretty fancy-sounding process—Chairside Economical Restoration of Esthetic Ceramic. Now say that five times fast! But don't worry if you can't because CEREC refers to a process where the dentist uses a patented computer-assisted technology to make a ceramic dental filling. The dentist first takes a three-dimensional (3-D) photograph of the prepared cavity. This image is then stored in the computer, which uses 3-D CAD/CAM software to refine the 3-D digital model. (CAD is the acronym for Computer Aided Design and CAM is the acronym for Computer Aided Manufacturing.)

Once the software has analyzed the cavity size and approximated the shape of the tooth and filling needed, a milling machine, controlled by the computer software, carves a finished restoration from a solid ceramic block. The filling is refined, fitted, the occlusion is adjusted, and then finally it's bonded/cemented to the tooth just like an indirect composite, inlay, or onlay would be. The big difference is that you get the equivalent of an indirect composite in just one visit to the dental office.

The CEREC system was developed in 1987 and in the hands of a skilled dentist, there's no doubt that the latest generation of composites and CEREC ceramics are far superior to amalgam fillings—and are a very safe filling material. The development of composite material, both direct and indirect, and the CEREC system of tooth restoration, makes the ADA's argument that amalgam is a better filling material impossible to sustain.

CEREC is truly an example of space age dentistry with the additional advantage of having a harder, better-fitting, and longer-lasting filling than amalgams or direct composites. Also, X-rays can penetrate a CEREC crown, allowing the dentist to see what is underneath. This is useful for detecting redecay or determining if any amalgam was left behind. Plus, CEREC has the advantage of being free of Bis-GMA. To date, not all dental offices have the CEREC system.

Metal-Free Dentistry

Some holistic dentists don't believe in using metal for any dental restoration, including metal onlays, crowns, and bridges (most onlays and crowns used today are gold or other metal alloys). Today, the most prevalent material used in metal-free dentistry is based on the same composite material that's used for fillings, but reinforced with interspersed translucent fibers. When these fibers have been added to a composite, it can be as strong as the traditional porcelain-to-metal crown (described later in the chapter), and has the added advantage of being an excellent replacement for metal crowns and onlays.

Many metal-free dentists believe that any metal dental restoration, aside from being a possible allergen, will interfere with the normal flow of energy along the body's meridians. This belief is based on an eastern philosophy of healing that says that every organ and every part of the body is directly linked to a specific tooth via meridians, or energy highways. Not everyone will exhibit a health problem directly related to having metals in their teeth, but those who are very sensitive, or whose health has been severely compromised, will be more susceptible.

At the date of publication, metal-free dentistry is still relatively new and the life expectancy of metal-free onlays, crowns, and bridges is still unknown. However, one of the positive aspects of this approach to restoring teeth is that the restorations can be easily repaired.

Gold

Gold restorations can be used for inlays, onlays, or crowns and are often used to replace mercury fillings when a comparable composite filling wouldn't be strong enough to restore the tooth for an extended period of time. In its elemental "pure" form, 24-carat gold is far too soft to be used for dental restorations. So what you think of as a "gold crown" is always alloyed with other metals such as copper, silver, platinum, palladium, cobalt, nickel, titanium, chromium, or zinc. If it's done properly and well cared for, a gold restoration can last 20, 30, 40 years and beyond.

Placing gold restorations requires at least two dental visits. Once the amalgam filling has been removed, the tooth is prepared and an impression is taken and sent to a dental laboratory where the restoration can be manufactured. It then takes another office appointment to check for proper fit and to permanently cement the restoration.

Numerous brands of gold filling materials are available. People who are sensitive to metals found in gold crowns, particularly nickel, can usually best tolerate materials that contain the highest percentage of gold and less of an allergenic metal. If you do choose a gold restoration, the amount of metal that is abraded from it will determine how much metal you'll be exposed to. For example, those who grind their teeth and have abrasive diets will abrade more. No matter how much it is stimulated and heated, however, neither the gold, nor any of the other materials found in it, will be released as a vapor.

For the majority of people, the small amount of abraded particles from a gold crown won't create an allergic issue. But if you know you're sensitive to any of the above-mentioned metals, especially nickel, tell your dentist and request a filling material that's free of them. For those who are prone to allergies, the Clifford Biocompatibility Test will be helpful in selecting the right material.

Porcelain-to-Metal and Porcelain Crowns

Porcelain crowns consist primarily of the same materials as glass—silicon and oxygen. The most commonly used porcelain restoration is porcelain fused to metal, or porcelain-to-metal. Aluminum, titanium, potassium, sodium, calcium and other oxides are often added to porcelain to give it strength and allow it to better fuse with the underlying metal. The main advantage of porcelain is that it's aesthetically pleasing—it's the restoration of choice for people who wish to have their dental crown restorations look as natural as possible.

Pure porcelain crowns are not fused to an underlying metal crown and are far more brittle than porcelain-to-metal or ceramic and gold crowns and onlays, which makes them more susceptible to fracturing or chipping. As a result, pure porcelain is generally only used for capping/crowning the front teeth. But with the advent of new composite materials, porcelain restorations can often be inexpensively repaired.

As with gold crowns, it usually takes two dental visits to prepare the tooth, take an impression, have the crown made at the lab, and then cemented. Since porcelain is harder than the tooth's enamel, it can, under certain conditions, cause the opposing natural tooth (or teeth) to wear down more quickly than normal. But if they're placed correctly, and taken care of, these fillings have a long life expectancy.

Titanium

Recently, titanium has become available for implant, inlay, and onlay restorations. While it doesn't have the same characteristics of gold, it is similar in terms of durability, the number of appointments required, and the cost. One drawback is aesthetics—the material is a grayish color. So far, titanium isn't a commonly used dental restorative material.

Safety of Dental Materials

I don't believe that any dental material will be 100 percent safe for everyone. At this point all we can do is work with what's available and choose the best, safest dental composite material. To date, my research hasn't uncovered any reason for the vast majority of the population to be concerned about composites. But I will continue to explore the latest findings and keep you updated on my website.

Although all evidence indicates that the percentage of people who could have a composite-related health issue is extremely small, anyone with numerous allergies, immune system issues, or breast cancer or a risk factor for it should consider using indirect composites. If you are in this category, I recommend using the Clifford Biocompatibility Test to help determine the most compatible dental material for you. I'd also recommend the Clifford test for anyone who is pregnant or nursing and wants to replace an amalgam filling.

Dental Material Biocompatibility Test

No discussion about replacing mercury fillings would be complete without discussing the biocompatibility of the replacement filling material. Biocompatibility means that a substance is compatible with the body and won't cause an allergic reaction. I recommend that everyone who is having their mercury fillings removed and replaced consider taking a biocompatibility test. As of 2008, over 2,000 different dental materials are in use, and no dental material is 100 percent safe for everyone. This means that you may be sensitive to a number of dental materials and it's impossible to guess which ones you may have a reaction to.

Unlike a food allergy, which can be readily removed from the diet, a dental filling is in your tooth 24 hours a day. Fillings that can be abraded or etched are a bigger concern than cements or cavity liners that are placed under a filling and have minimal exposure to the oral environment.

Biocompatibility testing is especially important for those who have numerous symptoms related to chronic mercury poisoning or other serious health conditions—especially immune system disorders. This group includes those with allergies or multiple sensitivities, whether they're dietary, chemical, or environmental.

If you decide to take the biocompatibility test, the most important consideration is time. Ask your dentist to order the test four to five weeks prior to your treatment appointment, if possible. Your dentist needs adequate time to analyze the test results and order the appropriate dental material for you, and it can easily take two to three weeks from the day the test is ordered to when the dentist receives the results.

If you choose *not* to have a biocompatibility test, your mercury safe dentist won't be able to guarantee the dental materials he or she selects will be compatible with you. In this situation, ask your dentist to select the materials shown to be the *most* compatible for the *greatest* number of patients. Mercury safe and holistic dentists are much more likely to be aware of the importance of biocompatibility testing and will be better able to advise you on appropriate replacement materials. The Clifford Biocompatibility Test is available to help dentists assess which dental materials are the most biocompatible for their patients. A dentist or health professional must order this test for you. (See Appendix D for more information on the test.)

Some holistic dentists may recommend muscle testing, also referred to as applied kinesiology, to determine which filling material is the most biocompatible. Typically with muscle testing, you'd hold the substance being tested in one hand and extend your opposite arm out parallel to the floor. The tester then puts downward pressure on your arm, and if the substance you are holding is biocompatible, the muscle will be able to resist the downward pressure. But if it isn't compatible, the muscle becomes weak and cannot resist the pressure, and the extended arm is easily pushed down.

Amalgam Filling Removal Sequence

Every mercury safe dentist agrees that mercury fillings should be safely removed, but this agreement doesn't always extend to which ones should be removed first, how many can be removed during one appointment, and in what order they should be removed. Some mercury safe dentists believe that the largest filling should be removed first. Others use a special Electro-Dermal-Screening (EDS) device, or similar devices, to evaluate the energetic (acupuncture) pathways to determine the electrical current of each filling and remove the one with the highest negative reading first. Most mercury safe dentists don't have this type of device, however, and in some states it isn't accepted.

There are also dentists who believe it's best to remove amalgam fillings by quadrant, starting with the quadrant that contains the largest and greatest number of amalgam fillings. (The mouth is divided into four quadrants, two in the upper jaw and two in the lower, with each quadrant containing eight teeth.) And some say it doesn't really matter which amalgams, or how many, are removed at each visit, as long as they're all removed as soon as possible.

Based on my research, no clear, compelling, and objective scientific evidence has surfaced to support one removal system over another. This isn't to validate or invalidate any of them, but to say that every patient is unique and the best approach is to have your mercury safe dentist explain to your satisfaction his or her view of the recommended removal sequence. My personal preference, unless there are compelling reasons not to, is to remove the largest amalgam first, or the ones closest to a gold crown.

But remember that ultimately the purpose of removing these fillings is to eliminate the source of your exposure to mercury from amalgam fillings. While there are exceptions, in my opinion the order in which they're removed isn't as important as removing them in the safest and quickest way possible.

Mercury Allergy

It's very important to consider your current state of health and past dental history when dealing with the removal of mercury fillings. For example, if you suspect you're among the 2 to 35 percent (or more) of the population who are allergic to mercury, you'll particularly benefit from spreading the removal process out over time. Or if you've experienced any problems after amalgam removal, it's possible your immune system is so depleted that it can't protect you from even the relatively small amount of mercury released during the safe removal procedure. If this has been your experience, you'll need to consider spreading amalgam removal over an extended period of time.

If you're concerned about a mercury allergy, have multiple environmental, chemical, or dietary allergies/sensitivities, or if you know that your immune system has been weakened, I recommend that you consider the MELISA® test (Memory Lymphocyte Immuno Stimulation Assay). This is a blood test specifically designed to test for sensitivity to metals, including mercury. You'll find more information about the MELISA® test in Appendix A.

Time Between Dental Visits

Even within the mercury safe dental community there is no consensus regarding how long you should wait between amalgam removal appointments. Some recommend waiting from six to eight weeks after the first removal appointment. Others believe that if you didn't have a problem when the first one or two fillings were removed, you can proceed with the removal and replacement procedure quickly.

Based on my experience, if you're in good health, aren't allergic to mercury, and can deal with the physical and psychological stress of removing the fillings, you can have your amalgam fillings removed as quickly as your mercury safe dentist recommends. However, if you don't fit into this category, talk to your mercury free dentist and consider spreading out the appointments over a longer period of time.

Last But Not Least

While it's important to weigh a filling's longevity and aesthetics with its biocompatibility and safety, any dental restorative material available today is infinitely safer than a mercury amalgam filling. You can find plenty of long-lasting and safe alternatives to amalgam, so I believe you should not let anything stop you from getting those toxic fillings removed! Mercury safe dentists are much more likely to stay up to date on the new and better replacement materials, so ask them to explain the advantages and disadvantages of each material.

What's Next

Not everyone will be able to have their mercury amalgam fillings removed as quickly as they would like to, and may have to spread their removal out over time. If you find yourself in this situation, all is not lost—there are steps you can take to minimize your exposure to mecury vapor while the fillings are still in your teeth. The next chaper will tell you how.

Ten

Reducing Mercury Exposure from Amalgam (Silver) Fillings

Based on what you've learned so far it's understandable that you may want to have all of your toxic mercury fillings removed as soon as possible. But that may not be feasible, for any number of reasons, that we covered in the previous chapter. So the issue is how to minimize the amount of mercury released from the fillings you have until you can start the safe removal process.

Two main actions stimulate the release of mercury vapor from amalgam fillings—disrupting the oxide layer that thinly covers their surface and heating the filling. In most cases, the two happen simultaneously. For example, many common actions will remove the microscopically thin oxide layer and heat the filling at the same time, such as brushing, eating, chewing gum, and tooth grinding.

The amount of mercury vapor released when an amalgam filling is heated is determined by the type, intensity, and length of stimulation, and whether it has a high or low copper content. (High copper amalgams release up to 50 times more mercury than low copper ones.) Mercury vapor release is highest while the filling is being actively stimulated. Once the stimulation stops, it gradually decreases, but the filling still releases mercury vapor for up to 90 minutes. The following are the most common methods of stimulation, along with recommendations for reducing the amount of mercury released. I've listed them in order of importance.

Tooth Grinding

It's estimated that 90 percent of the population grind their teeth at some time during their lives, and as many as 20 percent grind them extensively and continuously. Tooth grinding dramatically increases the release of mercury vapor from amalgam fillings by both disrupting the oxide layer and dramatically heating the fillings. Of course, the extent of tooth grinding, and thus the amount of mercury vapor released, varies from person to person. This will depend on:

- the number and size of the fillings

- whether or not the bite allows for a direct tooth-to-filling or filling-to-filling contact

- the intensity and duration of the grinding

Since the majority of tooth grinders do most of their grinding at night, mercury vapor release will take place for many hours, exposing the body to high levels of mercury during this period. While non-grinders get a respite from mercury exposure during sleep, tooth grinders receive their highest dose of mercury during this time. A tooth grinder with only a few amalgam fillings can release significantly more mercury than a person who has many more amalgams but doesn't grind. More mercury is released during tooth grinding than at any other time, except when amalgam fillings are placed, removed, or polished.

Recommendation

If you're a tooth grinder and need to delay having your mercury amalgam fillings removed, ask your dentist to make you a soft night-guard to prevent tooth-to-filling or filling-to-filling contact. If the delay in removing your fillings will be longer than a year, ask for a more durable, longer-lasting night-guard. Using a night-guard will significantly reduce your mercury vapor exposure and can also help relieve muscular stress and tension caused by grinding. Some people don't know if they grind their teeth, but if you're unsure, speak to your dentist about it, as he or she will be able to determine if you do.

Chewing Gum

Chewing gum increases the amount of mercury vapor released from amalgam fillings by up to 54 percent when compared to non-chewers. The key factor here is time—the longer you do anything that stimulates the release of mercury vapor, the more will be released. Other factors being equal, a frequent gum chewer who has a few amalgam fillings will be exposed to much more mercury vapor each day than a person who has more fillings but doesn't chew gum. The total amount of mercury released depends on how long, how often, and how vigorously the gum is chewed.

Recommendation

Simple answer. Don't chew gum until *all* your mercury fillings have been removed and replaced.

Brushing

Brushing your amalgam fillings, especially with a hard toothbrush and abrasive toothpaste, can increase mercury vapor levels in the mouth to more than 10 times the amount that some regulatory agencies allow in the workplace. The actual amount released is determined by the hardness of the bristles, how often you brush, the pressure used, and the duration of brushing.

The amount of mercury vapor released also depends on whether you use an electric or manual toothbrush. When used for the same amount of time, an electric toothbrush will stimulate the release of more mercury vapor than a manual one. This is because the bristles on an electric toothbrush are usually harder and generate many more strokes per minute. Thus, even if you use an electric toothbrush for a shorter period of time, the total amount of mercury released from the brushed fillings will still be significantly higher than from manual brushing.

Recommendation

You don't need to be concerned about decay developing on the surface of an amalgam filling, but it can develop at the margins where the filling meets the tooth. Until your mercury fillings are removed, brush the margins of your filling (where it meets with the tooth) lightly and quickly, and avoid brushing all other surfaces of the filling. Rinsing with room-temperature water after brushing to cool down the fillings will help minimize the amount of mercury released.

Clenching

While clenching doesn't appreciably heat amalgam fillings, it can cause an increase in mercury vapor release if this action brings a gold filling into continuous contact, or proximity, with an amalgam filling. For example, if you have a gold crown on an upper tooth and clenching brings it into direct contact with an amalgam filling on the lower opposing tooth, a battery-like effect called a "galvanic current" can result. This current can cause the release of high levels of mercury, even though the amalgam filling isn't being heated. The current can exist even if the teeth are not in contact, but the closer the two different types of fillings are to each other, the more powerful the current—resulting in the release of more mercury vapor.

Recommendation
If you know you're a clencher and have gold fillings in contact or proximity with amalgam fillings (ask your dentist if you're not sure), use a night-guard until the amalgam fillings are safely removed.

Hot Liquids and Foods

Drinking hot liquids and eating hot foods can significantly heat amalgam fillings and increase the release of mercury vapor. This form of filling stimulation is significant for people who drink large amounts of hot coffee or other hot beverages throughout the day.

Recommendation
This is easier said than done, but until your amalgams have been removed, it's best to cool liquids and foods to room-temperature, or rinse your mouth with room temperature water as soon as possible after eating or drinking.

Snacking

Snacking throughout the day heats the fillings by the abrasion/heating effects of chewing, consequently increasing the release of mercury vapor. The amount released depends on the number of snacks per day and how long the snacking lasts.

Recommendation
Don't snack between meals until your amalgams are removed, unless you have special dietary requirements, or eat foods that don't require chewing, such as juices, smoothies, or pureed foods.

Chewing Abrasive Foods

Chewing any food will heat amalgam fillings and stimulate the release of mercury. But abrasive foods such as nuts and seeds are more likely to do so because they easily disrupt the oxide layer, erode more amalgam particles from the fillings, and quickly heat the fillings to a higher temperature.

Recommendation

Avoid abrasive foods until your fillings are removed. If abrasive foods are an essential part of your diet, you can minimize the amount of chewing by grinding nuts and seeds in a blender or food processor or using nut/seed butters.

Cleaning and Polishing Amalgams at the Dental Office

Many dental offices use a cavitron or other ultrasonic cleaner to clean teeth. During an ultrasonic dental cleaning, heat is generated due to friction created between the tooth and the ultrasonic waves emitted from the cleaning tip. These instruments are routinely used in many dental offices to clean teeth and, if used on amalgam surfaces, can significantly increase the temperature of the fillings, which in turn can dramatically increase the amount of mercury vapor released.

Recommendation

Ask your dentist or dental hygienist not to use an ultrasonic cleaning device on the surfaces of your amalgam fillings. Handheld cleaning instruments can be used selectively in the margin areas, minimizing the amount of heat generated during cleaning. It's also important not to have the surfaces of your amalgam fillings polished after cleaning, as polishing dramatically heats the filling and increases the release of mercury vapor and amalgam particles. (Not using an ultrasonic cleaner on amalgams will also help minimize the dental hygienist's exposure to mercury vapor.)

Acidic Foods and Drinks

Acidic foods and drinks such as citrus fruits, pickles, sauerkraut, tomatoes, mustard, vinegar, acidic fruit juices, and soft drinks can etch the surfaces of amalgam fillings and cause the release of elemental mercury.

Recommendation

Limit consumption of these items until your amalgam fillings have been removed. If you must drink acidic beverages, use a straw, as it will keep the acidic liquid away from the fillings. Always remember to rinse your mouth with water after consuming acidic drinks and food.

Hot Baths and Saunas

Anything that increases the temperature of the oral cavity will heat your fillings and increase the amount of mercury vapor they release.

Recommendation

Hot baths and saunas have great value. If you enjoy them, you can keep your fillings cool by rinsing your mouth with room-temperature water every 5–10 minutes or so.

Smoking

Smoking can increase the temperature in the mouth during inhalation and, consequently, increase the amount of mercury vapor released. Although the amount released can be small, be aware of this fact if you smoke. Smoking also has a more direct and harmful effect on the immune system by increasing your exposure to cadmium, another very toxic heavy metal. Many symptoms of chronic cadmium poisoning are similar to those of chronic mercury poisoning. By placing additional stress on the immune system, smoking can reduce your body's ability to eliminate mercury.

Recommendation

If you're a smoker, I highly recommend that you seriously consider stopping.

Rinsing with Cool Water

Regardless of the type of stimulation, you can reduce your exposure to mercury vapor by always rinsing your mouth with room-temperature water after any activity that increases the fillings' temperature. It will be more effective if you leave the water in contact with the fillings for at least 30 seconds or so.

If you spit out the water after rinsing instead of swallowing it, you'll also remove mercury that's mixed with saliva. Not swallowing it will prevent any elemental mercury from being transformed into organic or methyl mercury in the mouth or intestine.

Following these recommendations can significantly reduce your exposure to mercury vapor while your amalgam fillings are still in your teeth. But *please*, don't be lulled into thinking that the above precautions will eliminate your need to have these poisonous fillings removed.

What's Next?

Similarly, don't be lulled into thinking that once you've had your amalgams removed you're all done. Your body still needs to purge itself of the accumulated mercury, and you can help it do that with a mercury detoxification program. Read on to learn about the next step that can help to put you back on the road to optimum health.

Eleven

Mercury Detoxification

Mercury detoxification is a big subject and I've written an entire book about it: *Mercury Detoxification: The Natural Way to Remove Mercury from Your Body*. Since that book covers the subject extensively, in this chapter I'll just introduce the concepts and principles involved in supporting your body's efforts at removing accumulated mercury. If you want to learn more, head over to my website, www.dentalwellness4u.com, where you can purchase a copy.

Mercury is wily. Its vapor sneaks out of amalgam fillings all too easily, then enters into and accumulates throughout the body. Your body does its best to remove it, but if enough mercury accumulates it can overwhelm the body's immune system. That means you have to help your body fight this poisonous substance by participating in a *mercury detoxification program*—a program specifically designed to support the body's effort to remove mercury and help heal the damage.

My program explains the process of mercury detoxification, what you need to know about vitamins and nutritional supplements, and how you can support the detoxification process with treatments such as sweat therapy, colonics, and lymphatic stimulation. It explains what you can do to support intestinal and brain health, teaches you how to monitor your program, explains the use of pharmaceutical chelators, and discusses the common tests for mercury.

Plus it provides innovative and easy-to-use charts to keep track of the supplements and other products I recommend. It will serve as your A to Z guide to mercury detoxification.

The Steps that Need to Be Taken

You need to take three critically important steps to successfully treat chronic mercury poisoning, and each one is an essential part of any mercury detoxification program. You'll need to remove the source of the exposure, support your body's efforts at removing the accumulated mercury, and provide it with what it needs to repair the damage done by mercury.

You're now well aware now of how damaging mercury is to your health. That's the bad news. But the good news is that the body is truly miraculous. Intelligently supported, it can be very effective at removing mercury and reversing, as much as possible, the damage that has been done. So don't waste time dwelling on the negative aspects of chronic mercury poisoning. Instead, focus on the fact that you've discovered a major contributor to your health problems and know you can do something positive about it.

Why Participate in a Mercury Detoxification Program

Your decision to participate in a mercury detoxification program should be based on the following criteria. You want to improve:

- your overall health
- symptoms that are directly and indirectly related to chronic mercury poisoning
- your immune/detoxification system
- your resistance to toxins, infections, allergies, and other more serious diseases
- your quality of life and your life expectancy

There are two evaluations, subject and objective, that will help you determine if a mercury detoxification program will benefit you.

Subjective Evaluation: Taking a Good Look at Yourself

Subjective evaluation involves assessing your own symptoms and health issues and determining if they're related to chronic mercury poisoning. For example, if you have, or had, amalgam fillings and find you also have a number of symptoms or diseases related to chronic mercury poisoning, you should very seriously consider participating in a detoxification program. (Refer back to Chapter 5: "Symptoms and Diseases Related to Chronic Mercury Poisoning" for a list of the more common symptoms and diseases.)

Objective Evaluation: Testing for Mercury

Objectively evaluating the level of your mercury exposure requires testing. There are a number of tests for mercury, including hair, blood, fecal, and urine. (Refer to Appendix A: "Testing for Mercury" for information about each test.) Based on my experience, the fecal metals test and the urine mercury challenge (or provoked) test are the best for providing a general indication of the extent of your mercury toxicity. These objective and scientific tests are also beneficial if you have any doubt about whether or not your body has accumulated mercury from your amalgam fillings. Correctly interpreted, the fecal metals test can also be helpful in monitoring your mercury detoxification program. (I believe many pro-amalgam dentists will read my book and I strongly encourage them to have a fecal metals test done. If they do, I doubt they will ever again support the use of amalgam fillings.)

The Confusion about Mercury Detoxification

While health practitioners and the mercury safe dental community agree about the need for safe amalgam removal, there's considerably less agreement about the most effective way to support your body's efforts to remove the accumulated mercury.

You'll find programs either suggesting very few or too many supplements, and those recommending very low dosages or very high dosages. Still others think the only way to detoxify mercury is with pharmaceutical chelators without using any supplements.

This lack of a clear consensus can be confusing, especially when the fundamentals of mercury detoxification haven't been adequately explained and understood. There is no doubt, if you don't have enough information, you won't be able to make an informed choice regarding mercury detoxification. It was in response to the need for clarity that I developed a safe and natural approach to mercury detoxification.

A Natural Approach

My program approaches mercury detoxification in the safest and most natural way possible. By taking the approach that you don't have to get sick to get well, using natural products, starting with low dosages, and moving slowly, undesirable side effects will be avoided. The goal of my program is to support—and ultimately improve—your body's own extraordinary ability to effectively remove stored mercury.

Most people aren't aware that the body has the ability to remove mercury. But if the mercury exposure is chronic and excessive, the body becomes less and less able to do so. Thus, if you don't provide your body with the supplements it needs to remove the accumulated mercury and heal the damage done, it won't be able to do its job. Once your body's ability to remove mercury has been restored and your mercury levels have been significantly reduced, the program can continue to function as a health maintenance program. In other words, it's designed to not only help eliminate mercury, but to also help you achieve an optimal state of health—and then keep you healthy.

How Effective Will it Be?

While the basics of mercury detoxification are the same for everyone, each person's situation is unique and should be dealt with accordingly. All of the following must be taken into consideration when evaluating how effective a mercury detoxification program will be and how soon you can expect results:

- the present state of your oral and overall health

- your diet and supplement program

- the health of your immune/antioxidant system

- the extent and duration of your exposure to mercury

- your body's ability to eliminate mercury

Everyone who has or had amalgam fillings is mercury toxic to some degree. As you know, the extent of your toxicity depends on many factors, and this will vary from person to person. When evaluating the length of a mercury detoxification program, the sum of these factors will help determine how long you should participate in the program and the benefits you'll receive from it. I've created a simple risk evaluation model to help determine your exposure to mercury and you can take it by going to my website, www.dentalwellness4u.com, and clicking on "Mercury Risk Evaluation" in the Frequently Asked Questions (FAQ) section on the homepage.

Except for the possible use of a medically supervised pharmaceutical chelator, everything in my program is either naturally produced by the body, required by the body but must be obtained from outside sources (e.g. vitamin C), or is an accepted health-supporting nutrient. All the supplements and nutrients used in my program are sold on my website, over the counter at health food stores, and by many online vitamin companies. None require a prescription, but if you have multiple mercury related symptoms, or more serious health issues that could be related to chronic mercury poisoning, I highly recommend that you consult with a qualified health professional.

A Safe Approach to Mercury Detoxification

Another important aspect of a mercury detoxification program is its safety. My philosophy is that it's not necessary to get sick while trying to get well. Because some people detoxify rapidly—even too quickly in some cases—I believe that you should always *start low* and *go slow*. Detoxifying from mercury too rapidly can be difficult and uncomfortable for some and may cause numerous unwanted symptoms, such as headaches, nausea, and diarrhea.

Some detoxification programs recommend supplements in dosages that may be too high for some people. This can result in unwanted side effects that could either stir up more toxins than their bodies can effectively eliminate, or their immune system is too depleted to handle a more aggressive approach. Others may experience an allergic reaction to some detoxification products, or have undesirable reactions to pharmaceutical chelators that the body couldn't handle.

The safe, natural, slow, and gentle approach that I promote is even more important for those who are very mercury toxic, whose immune systems have been severely compromised, and those who may have difficulty with rapid detoxification. Because their health is so fragile, they may not be able to handle an aggressive approach to detoxification, and it is imperative that they seek counsel from a qualified health practitioner.

Because my program covers every aspect of mercury detoxification, it provides a sound foundation that can be built on or even reduced, as the case may be. It's also designed to let you become more involved in deciding what supplements and what dosages you should take. After all, it's your body, and your body will quickly tell you how well it can handle what you are putting into it, regardless of what I or anyone else tells you should or shouldn't happen. So it's important that you listen carefully to what it is telling you.

Tolerance Testing

I utilize tolerance testing to determine how well the body can tolerate the supplements and nutritional products necessary to eliminate mercury and begin to heal the damage done by it. I do this by introducing supplements and nutritional products slowly, and in low dosages, to prevent or minimize any undesirable side effects that could occur if the initial dose was too high. The two most commonly seen side effects of taking high doses of nutritional supplements are allergic and dose-related reactions. Supplements that are made by the body or needed from outside sources shouldn't cause allergic reactions. But dose-related reactions, even with substances the body normally wouldn't be allergic to, can occur if the dosage is excessive. The old adage "too much of a good thing" applies here.

Intestinal Support

The small and large intestine play an important and complex role in overall health, and especially in detoxification. When the body releases mercury into the intestine from the common bile duct, it is *technically* considered to be out of the body. But it still has to travel 26 feet through the intestine before it can be considered *officially* removed. During that journey a lot of things can happen to it. Bottom line, unless the intestine is properly supported with the use of fiber and supplements that help prevent the re-absorption of mercury back into the body, all of the mercury that passes into the intestine may not actually get out of it!

Brain Support

Mercury is classified as a neurotoxin. A neurotoxin is a toxic substance that inhibits, damages, or destroys the tissues of the brain and central nervous system. Many of the short and long-term symptoms related to chronic mercury poisoning are neurological, so supporting brain health can substantially improve the success of a mercury detoxification program.

I've devoted a special section to brain support in my *Mercury Detoxification* book, and it's a must-read for anyone with any neurological symptoms related to chronic mercury poisoning. It should be noted that the neurological damage done by chronic mercury poisoning isn't restricted to physical symptoms. Chronic mercury poisoning can cause or contribute to numerous emotional and psychological symptoms, such as depression, anxiety, mood swings, memory loss, brain fog, and irritability. You can review the neurological symptoms related to chronic mercury poisoning in Chapter 5: "Symptoms and Diseases Related to Chronic Mercury Poisoning."

Apoptosis: Cellular Death and Mercury Detoxification

To be successful, a mercury detoxification program must consider the consequences of cellular death. It's estimated that *each day* billions of cells in the body die, and approximately the same number of new cells are created. Approximately every 7 years, every cell in the general body will be replaced. (The cells in the brain are an exception—when brain cells die, new ones aren't created.)

Apoptosis (a-pop-toe-sis) describes cellular death from something other than an accident (such as a fall) or another form of external trauma. It's what takes place when a cell dies of old age, is damaged beyond repair by toxins and poisons, is starved of vital nutrients, or has been compromised in such an extreme way that the health of other cells is threatened. Some refer to this process as "cellular suicide." Regardless of the cause, when a cell dies it breaks into billions of pieces that the body, in its infinite wisdom, recognizes as debris and cleans up. The body then "reuses" the salvageable cellular components to help make new cells and, if possible, will try to dispose of what it doesn't need.

Apoptosis is a relatively new field with much still to be learned. But my research shows that we need to ask some important questions about apoptosis in regards to chronic mercury poisoning and mercury detoxification. Those questions are:

- Where does the mercury inside a cell go when it dies and is broken up?

- How does the body deal with it?

- Does the mercury have access to other cells, or to the new cells that are being created?

- Does it stay attached to proteins and enzymes?

- Can it escape its existing attachment seeking other places to attach to?

An even more important question revolves around what happens to the mercury in *brain cells* that die. The brain doesn't generate new cells and this could mean that if the brain doesn't have sufficient amounts of mercury chelating antioxidants, all of the mercury released from dead brain cells can't be captured and removed. The possibility exists that other cells in the brain will absorb the released mercury. This suggests that even if the brain is no longer exposed to external sources of mercury, such as from amalgam fillings, the viable brain cells will still have to deal with the mercury released from dead brain cells. This re-absorption into other brain cells could account for the fact that it takes longer for neurologically related symptoms to improve.

A similar situation exists with mercury released from dead cells into the cells of the general, or systemic, body. If the body doesn't have adequate amounts of glutathione (GSH) and alpha lipoic acid (ALA) to capture the released mercury, it could find its way into existing cells and the new ones that are constantly being created. The main difference here is that, unlike in the brain, the body can replace the damaged or dead cells.

In my research, I haven't found any studies that deal with these concerns. So until we know more, the best preventive approach is to eliminate every source of mercury exposure and commit to a mercury detoxification program designed to support the body's efforts to remove mercury. At the end of this chapter I'll discuss NCD, a product that I believe can support the body's ability to deal with the mercury released from dead cells and, if you still have amalgams, help remove the mercury still entering the body.

Monitoring Your Mercury Detoxification Program

Monitoring your mercury detoxification program, both objectively and subjectively, can be very helpful in assessing its progress. The body is a miracle in how it can repair itself, if given the support it needs. And it's very good about letting you know how it's doing. Thus, monitoring is an essential component of any mercury detoxification program. (You'll find detailed information on monitoring, including helpful charts for recording and monitoring your improvement, in my book *Mercury Detoxification*.)

What Does the Body Need?

Antioxidants have the crucial task of removing mercury and other heavy metals from the body and neutralizing free radicals and toxins. But they don't come from thin air; the body manufactures them from amino acids. But when it has been overwhelmed by chronic mercury exposure, the body won't be able to produce enough GSH and ALA to keep up with what is being lost.

Ensuring that your body gets the materials it needs to manufacture antioxidants is the only way to be certain it will be able to protect you. This point is particularly important if your exposure to mercury has occurred over a long period of time, because the body will be seriously deficient in these critically important antioxidants. So the bottom line is that people who take the right supplements, in appropriate amounts, will be the most successful at removing stored mercury.

Mercury Cannot Be Detoxified!

The term "mercury detoxification" is commonly used to describe how the body removes mercury, but technically it isn't accurate. By definition, detoxification is the process the body uses to neutralize and eliminate toxins and other substances it wants to remove. Simply put, this process involves antioxidants transporting the toxin to the liver where it is broken down into water soluble, harmless compounds that can then be safely removed. Many types of antioxidants are involved in this process, including the body's most abundant one, glutathione (GSH). In the normal detoxification process, GSH may be damaged while doing its job, but it is then repaired and is able to continue its battle against the bad guys.

But this isn't the case when it comes to removing mercury. In the body, mercury can't be broken down or detoxified into anything except mercury. Thus, mercury must be "physically" escorted from the body by its primary mercury chelating antioxidants, glutathione and alpha lipoic acid. Remember, in removing mercury, these "escorts" are permanently lost and, over time, their levels will dramatically decrease.

Thus, the day you have your last mercury filling removed is also the day you'll be the most deficient in these mercury chelating antioxidants! While you will have eliminated the main source of mercury exposure, unless you've been supplementing during this time, your body's levels of GSH and ALA will be at their lowest. But it doesn't stop there. Removing your amalgam fillings doesn't mean the body will stop its efforts to remove mercury! Even after your amalgams have been removed, your body will continue to eliminate as much mercury as it possibly can. This means more and more GSH and ALA will be lost every minute of every day and you'll become even more susceptible to toxins, poisons, and free radicals.

While the body can manufacture antioxidants from the amino acids it gets from dietary protein, without your help it will never get enough from that source to restore what has been lost. Unless you give it what it needs via supplementation, the process of removing the stored mercury will take much longer. And any improvements in symptoms will be delayed accordingly.

Half-life of Mercury: True or False?

The term "half-life" applies to a material that's radioactive. For example, uranium-238 has a half-life of 4.5 billion years. So if you started with a pound of it on your kitchen table today, in 4.5 billion years you'd have eight ounces of it on your table. In another 4.5 billion years half of that would be gone, leaving four ounces on the table, and so on. It wouldn't matter if you put it in the freezer, buried it, or sent it to the moon, the decay process would continue unabated.

The idea of a half-life for mercury has been used to suggest how long it will take for mercury to leave the body. But what's important to understand is that *mercury from amalgam fillings is not radioactive, and does not have a half-life.* In fact, suggesting that mercury has a half-life is inaccurate and misleading.

That means the mercury that enters and accumulates in your body will not decay or just disappear over time. Yet, some people still refer to the half-life of mercury when talking about how long it will stay in the body. Mercury doesn't just miraculously vanish into thin air! I don't know how this misconception got started, but you can't simply wait for mercury to automatically disappear. It won't!

Symptom Improvement: What to Expect

I've been involved with mercury detoxification for over 30 years, and the question I hear most often is, "If I participate in a mercury detoxification program, when will the symptoms caused by mercury poisoning disappear?" It's a great question! After all, why would anyone want to expend the time, energy, and money and not see results? The answer has two parts. First, the time it takes for any improvement in symptoms related to chronic mercury poisoning depends on how much mercury has accumulated and the health of your immune system. Second, we know that once the source of mercury is removed, the body can repair the damage done to it when properly supported, if the harm done by mercury is reversible. Because brain cells cannot be replaced, some of the neurological damage done by mercury may not be reversible.

A number of studies have shown the improvements in symptoms and diseases related to chronic mercury poisoning both after amalgam fillings have been removed and when a detoxification program was included. These studies are very encouraging, and demonstrate how wonderfully the body can respond once the source of this poison has been removed and the body is supported in its efforts at removing mercury. Chapter 12: "Health Improvements Related to Amalgam Removal and Mercury Detoxification" discusses these studies.

All Detoxification Programs Aren't the Same

You'll find there are countless detoxification/cleansing/fasting programs offered. But they're not all the same. They range from liver detoxification to colon cleansing, from juice and water fasts to weight loss programs, just to name a few. While they may overlap in some areas, their focus is fundamentally different. If it isn't specifically called a *mercury detoxification program*, chances are it isn't designed to adequately support your body's efforts to remove mercury.

Essential Detoxification Supplements

My book *Mercury Detoxification* discusses the supplements needed to fully support a safe mercury detoxification program. Many supplements aren't directly involved in the removal of mercury but play a supportive role, either in protecting and repairing antioxidants or helping to heal the damage done by mercury. However, there are certain supplements and supportive products that I consider essential to the success of a mercury detoxification program. This isn't to say that you should only use these eight at the exclusion of the others in my program. No, my point is that without including these eight, I doubt you'll be able to achieve the results you are seeking. They are:

- N-Acetyl Cysteine (NAC)

- Alpha Lipoic Acid (ALA)

- Glutathione (GSH)

- Selenium (Se)

- Free Form Amino Acids

- Multiple Vitamin

- Multiple Mineral

- Vitamin C

I've learned that most people not only want the best quality products available, but to be able to access what they need from one source. In response—and because I consider these eight supplements so crucial—I developed my own supplement product line so I could be assured of the quality and purity of these supplements.

To accomplish this, I worked with one of the leading producers of hypoallergenic nutritional supplements. They follow the strict guidelines of Good Manufacturing Practices (GMP) and adhere to quality and purity standards of the U.S. Pharmacopeia (USP). All ingredients used are free of common allergens, including dairy, wheat, corn, soy, yeast, and gluten. No sugar, starch, maltodextrin, artificial sweeteners, colors, flavors, salicyates, or preservatives are used in these products.

I consider these supplements to be the best available. You can learn more and purchase these products by going to my website, www.dentalwellness4u. com, and selecting "Mercury Detoxification Supplements and Products" from the list of Frequently Asked Questions (FAQ). Detailed information about them is available on the website and in my mercury detoxification book.

Additional Supportive Products

NCD

NCD is a patented formula that utilizes the natural cleansing properties of zeolite. Zeolite is a natural volcanic mineral with a unique, complex crystalline structure. The honeycomb framework of cavities and channels (like cages) works at the cellular level to trap heavy metals and toxins. In fact, because it is a negatively charged mineral, zeolite acts as a magnet that draws positively charged toxins to it, capturing them in its cage and safely removing them from the body.

NCD is especially adept at capturing mercury atoms before they attach to proteins or enzymes, making it an important line of defense for those who still have their amalgam fillings, as well as for dentists and their staff who are continuously exposed to mercury at the office. My evaluation of the available research indicates that NCD can also play a beneficial role in protecting the body from the mercury released from cells that die and are broken apart.

Supplied in a liquid form, NCD is easily absorbed into the body from the intestine. In addition, it may also offer intestinal support by capturing mercury and other metals as they meet during their passage through the intestine. While it has long been known that zeolite has many other beneficial health-supporting qualities, in my opinion its ability to capture and remove harmful metals makes it a positive addition to a mercury detoxification program.

However, I found no evidence that NCD increases the production of glutathione, or other antioxidants, nor can it support the body's efforts at healing the damage done by mercury. As such, I consider it to be a valuable adjunct to my mercury detoxification program, but used on its own I don't believe it will yield the improvements in symptoms and diseases related to chronic mercury poisoning that you want to achieve. You'll find additional information about NCD, including how to order it, on my website, www.dentalwellness4u.com

Chlorella

Studies show that substances in chlorella can remove mercury in the body and intestine. It isn't known how chlorella does this, but it does contain cysteine, possibly allowing it to increase glutathione production and bind to mercury in the intestine. Chlorella is a food and its high concentration of vitamins, minerals, and digestible protein offer many other health benefits. Some people have problems digesting the cell membrane of chlorella, which can create unwanted gas and flatulence. Taking a digestive enzyme containing cellulase will often alleviate this problem. As with NCD, I consider it to be an important adjunct to my detoxification program.

What You Can Do

If you're considering participating in a mercury detoxification program, I recommend you read *Mercury Detoxification: The Natural Way to Remove Mercury from Your Body*. I wrote it because I couldn't find anything at the time that was written for the layperson and comprehensively covered this very important topic. For many, mercury detoxification is absolutely necessary to improve their health. It's also essential to have as much information as possible at hand when making a decision about participating in a mercury detoxification program.

Mercury Detoxification will show you how to support your body's efforts at removing mercury in the safest, most effective, and most natural way possible. If this is your first experience with a mercury detoxification program, it will act as your A to Z guide to this health-building process, and put all the elements needed into a single, accessible resource. It will also be beneficial if you made a previous attempt at detoxifying and didn't achieve the desired results. When it comes to eliminating mercury from the body, the more you know about the detoxification process, the better off you'll be. *Mercury Detoxification* explains:

- why removing mercury from your body is so important to your overall health

- how the detoxification process works

- the role and importance of the immune system in mercury detoxification

- what vitamin and nutritional supplements you need to support your body's efforts at removing mercury

- the importance of supporting intestinal health during this process

- the value and importance of providing your body with healing "brain food"

- how to tolerance test supplements to minimize potential side effects

- the role of pharmaceutical chelating agents in the detoxification process

- testing for mercury and how it can be used to effectively monitor your detoxification program

- how to use supplement schedule charts to track your program and make it exceptionally easy to follow

In a nutshell, *Mercury Detoxification* provides you with the information you need to understand and participate in a safe and effective mercury detoxification program. The book also provides you with an extensive reference section if you want to review the supporting science. You can read chapter excerpts and purchase it at www.dentalwellness4u.com.

What's Next

The next chapter introduces you to the improvements in symptoms experienced by those who had their fillings removed but didn't participate in a mercury detoxification program, and the improvements seen in those who did both.

Twelve

Health Improvements Related to Amalgam Removal and Mercury Detoxification

Everyone wants to be healthy and stay healthy. The vast majority of people I've spoken to who decided to remove their amalgam fillings wanted to know if their symptoms would improve after removal. In this chapter you'll be able to evaluate the improvement in symptoms and diseases between those who only had their amalgam fillings removed and those who also participated in a mercury detoxification program.

Amalgam Filling Removal and Symptom Improvement

In the largest collection of studies of its kind, Sam Ziff, a gifted researcher, compiled extensive data that verified improvement in symptoms related to chronic mercury poisoning—*after* the participants' amalgam fillings were removed and replaced. This extraordinary collection of studies is significant because of the large number of participants (1,569) and the extent of information it contains. The studies showed the following:

- symptom
- total number of symptoms
- number improved or cured
- percentage improved or cured
- percentage with symptom

If you're suffering from any of the symptoms listed in the chart below, you will find the column titled "Percentage Improved or Cured" very encouraging.

Symptom Improvement after Mercury Amalgam Filling Removal				
Symptom	Total # of Symptoms	# Improved or Cured	% Improved or Cured	% with Symptom
Lack of Energy	91	88	97	6
Metallic Taste	260	247	95	17
Gum Problems	129	121	94	8
Anxiety	96	80	93	5
Depression	347	315	91	22
Irritability	132	119	90	8
Allergy	81	68	89	14
Dizziness	343	301	88	22
Bloating	88	70	88	6
Chest Pains	79	69	87	5
Headaches	531	460	87	34
Irregular Heartbeat	159	139	87	10
Fatigue	705	603	86	45
Ulcers (Oral Cavity)	189	162	86	12
Nervousness	158	131	83	10
Muscle Tremor	126	104	83	8
Intestinal Problems	231	192	83	15

Symptom Improvement after Mercury Amalgam Filling Removal				
Symptom	*Total # of Symptoms*	*# Improved or Cured*	*% Improved or Cured*	*% with Symptom*
Numbness Anywhere	118	97	82	8
Lack of Concentration	270	216	80	17
Insomnia	187	146	78	12
Multiple Sclerosis	113	86	76	7
Memory Loss	265	193	73	17
Vision Problems	462	289	63	29
Blood Pressure Problems	99	53	54	6

In my opinion, the extent of improvement and the time it took to see results would be directly related to:

- how long the individual was mercury toxic
- the amount of damage mercury had done to the body and central nervous system
- the participant's overall health at the time of removal
- the health of the immune and detoxification systems, e.g., liver/kidneys

Ultimately, the importance of these studies is that the *actual and significant improvement* took place after the participants' mercury fillings were removed.

Health Observations Before and After Amalgam Removal

Another study with the same theme was done by a Swiss dentist, Dr. Paul Engel. In his classical study, *Health Observations Before and After Amalgam Removal*, he recorded a list of symptoms his patients expressed *prior* to having their fillings removed and then recorded the improvement in the same patients' symptoms *after* amalgam removal.

Dr. Engel's study began in the mid 1990s, and what makes his work so meaningful is that he was the dentist who originally placed the amalgam fillings of those participating in his study and was also the one who removed them. It's a distinct advantage to be able to track your own patients' symptoms over a long period of time, and then also be able to personally witness and record improvements in those symptoms.

Other than the supplements individual participants may have taken before or during the study, no one participated in a controlled mercury detoxification program. Fifty-two women and 23 men participated, and Dr. Engel evaluated 53 symptoms. These ranged from 36 complaints of migraine headaches to one case of diabetes. The following chart shows the 12 most common symptoms listed by participants prior to having their amalgams removed.

Symptoms Prior to Amalgam Removal			
Symptom	# of Complaints	Symptom	# of Complaints
Migraine	36	Allergies	13
Headache	32	Vision Disturbances	13
Gastrointestinal Problems	27	Back Pain	12
Neck Tensions	25	Mental Disorder	12
Paresthesia	19	Joint Pain	10
Dizziness	18	Shoulder/Arm Pain	10

After the amalgams were removed, each participant graded the changes in their health. Dr. Engel's study provides another example of how amalgam removal can, over time, significantly improve a number of symptoms directly related to chronic mercury poisoning.

Percent of Subjects Reporting Changes Due to Filling Removal	
Change Noted	%
Much Better	68
Better	12
Somewhat Better	9
No Improvement	7
Worse	1
No Assessment	3

Dr. Lichtenberg's Study

In another illuminating study, Dr. H. Lichtenberg studied 118 patients in his dental practice. He began the study in 1990 when he evaluated each participant for 38 symptoms and complaints commonly related to chronic mercury poisoning. The study consisted of 97 women and 21 men, ranging in age from 18 to 73. The average age of participants was 45, and 17 of the 38 symptoms listed were common to every participant. Four years after amalgam removal, all patients responded to an identical survey, with the following results:

- 48% of the symptoms were reduced

- 31% of the symptoms were eliminated

- 21% of the symptoms were unchanged

The following is a list of the 38 symptoms evaluated in the Lichtenberg study, the number of symptoms experienced prior to amalgam removal, the number reduced, and the number eliminated after removal. Symptoms are listed in alphabetical order.

A. Number experiencing symptoms before amalgam removal

B. Number whose symptoms were reduced after amalgam removal

C. Number whose symptoms were eliminated after amalgam removal

Lichtenberg Study Symptoms							
Symptoms	*A*	*B*	*C*	*Symptoms*	*A*	*B*	*C*
Allergy	65	40	3	Insomnia	54	31	13
Bad Breath	41	20	17	Irrational Fear	42	27	10
Bleeding Gums	50	19	25	Irritability	76	42	19
Blisters and Sores	46	20	21	Joint Pain	67	34	13
Bloating	69	33	18	Legs Cramps	39	16	19
Chest Pain	31	13	9	Metallic Taste	72	12	59
Cold Hands/Feet	58	20	18	Migraine	21	11	6
Constipation	44	22	7	Muscle Fatigue	73	33	14
Depression	56	34	16	Muscle Tremor	53	21	21
Diarrhea	48	23	20	Nasal Congestion	52	29	17
Dizziness	57	33	18	Nasal Discharge	32	14	13

Lichtenberg Study Symptoms							
Symptoms	A	B	C	Symptoms	A	B	C
Facial Tension	56	24	18	Poor Appetite	21	8	8
Fatigue	98	54	19	Poor Concentration	90	50	14
Frequent Infections	43	20	19	Poor Memory	77	41	13
Skin Reaction	51	28	10	Sciatic Pain	30	17	4
Headache	68	41	17	Tender Teeth	49	20	29
Heart Problems	25	11	6	Throat Irritation	67	31	24
Hunger Pain	60	22	14	Urinary Disorders	29	15	5
Intestinal Cramps	50	24	14	Watery Eyes	43	19	15

To me, what makes these three studies so fascinating is the clear message they send to patients and health practitioners about the improvement in symptoms related to chronic mercury poisoning—*after amalgam fillings were removed!*

These studies also send a clear message to pro-amalgam dentists. The mercury released from the supposedly "safe" and "harmless" amalgam fillings is poisoning their patients and contributing to a vast number of health symptoms related to chronic mercury poisoning. Even more importantly, these studies tell pro-amalgam dentists that they can have a positive influence on the health of their patients by safely removing these poisonous fillings and replacing them with safe restorations.

Pro-amalgam dentists can argue endlessly about the validity of these studies and say that anecdotal evidence isn't scientific proof. To those who feel this way, I recommend you talk to patients whose health improved after having their amalgam fillings removed. I guarantee they won't care about the ADA's opinion on the value of anecdotal evidence. While the ADA may not put any stock in subjective (direct human experience) studies because they can't be "scientifically" validated, those who have experienced an improvement in their health most certainly do.

Mercury Detoxification Programs and
Amalgam Removal: Related Health Improvements

As with the preceding studies, the following two support the link between health improvement and the removal of amalgam fillings. But even more, they show the link between health improvement, amalgam removal, *and participation in a mercury detoxification program.*

The first study, "Dental Amalgam and Health Experience: Exploring Health Outcomes and Issues for People Medically Diagnosed with Mercury Poisoning" by

Linda Jones (School of Psychology, Massey University, Wellington, New Zealand), evaluated 35 people who had previously been told that their symptoms were psychosomatic (including cognitive deficits and mood swings.) The most common complaints were chronic fatigue syndrome, candidiasis, allergies, migraines, and chronic or recurring flu symptoms—all of which are directly or indirectly related to chronic mercury poisoning.

Of the 32 participants who began amalgam removal, 29 (90 percent) reported enduring health gains. Of the 30 who completed both amalgam removal and a mercury detoxification program, 21 experienced a full return to health and the activities of daily life. Eight others in the study reported recovering from the symptoms they attributed to mercury, but now had either a new problem related to detoxification or a pre-existing condition that didn't improve. Only one person who followed the detoxification protocols experienced no lasting improvement. The three who hadn't begun amalgam removal were still ill and stated that their health was deteriorating.

The second study by Lindh and Associates looked at improvements in symptoms and the quality of life of 776 people who had their amalgam fillings removed and participated in a mercury detoxification program. The subjects previously suffered from an array of symptoms directly or indirectly related to chronic mercury poisoning, including those related to general, neurological, psychiatric and oral health. Although every symptom expressed wasn't eliminated, more than 70 percent of those who completed both amalgam removal and a detoxification program reported a substantial improvement and increased quality of life.

What These Studies Mean

Two things stand out in these studies. First, even if you only remove the major source of mercury exposure (amalgam fillings), improvements in related symptoms will be seen. Second, participating in a mercury detoxification program after amalgam removal can result in an even greater health improvement.

Safely removing these poisonous fillings and participating in a mercury detoxification program should be regarded as essential treatment for chronic mercury poisoning. Once you've had your amalgam fillings removed and participate in a mercury detoxification program, the improvements you'll experience will eventually tell you which symptoms were connected to chronic mercury poisoning.

Of course, mercury isn't the only cause of, or contributor to, your health problems, but it's one that you can identify and readily treat. And it's also clear that those who have symptoms related to chronic mercury poison and *do not* have their amalgams removed cannot expect those symptoms to improve.

What's Next

I've consulted with thousands of people about the health hazards of mercury amalgam (silver) fillings. Once they discover how the mercury vapor released from amalgams can harm their health, they ask the obvious question: "Why do dentists still use these poisonous fillings?" In my opinion the answer is directly connected to the ADA, which continues to advocate their safety and use in dentistry. In the next chapter, I'll discuss why the ADA does so and why I think it is absolutely wrong in defending the use of these poisonous fillings.

Thirteen

American Dental Association: Assessing the Blame

Let's review some key facts. First of all, there's complete agreement in the scientific community that mercury is a powerful poison. Secondly, there's *no safe level of mercury!* Even one atom of mercury in the body is doing harm. We know mercury is a powerful neurotoxin, is mutagenic, and can cause autism and other learning and developmental disorders. It passes through the placenta to the fetus and via breast milk to the nursing baby.

We also know that 50 percent of an amalgam (silver) filling is elemental mercury and releases toxic mercury vapor, 80 percent of which enters the body. Continuous exposure to mercury vapor from amalgam fillings will, over time, result in mercury accumulation in the body, contributing to or making worse every known health issue. These are the facts. But I don't believe the ADA wants you to know these facts.

It is either unaware of, or refuses to acknowledge, the thousands of studies that prove mercury is an extremely poisonous substance even in extraordinarily small amounts. In spite of the overwhelming scientific evidence, the ADA continues to assert that amalgam fillings are safe and harmless. And it continues to do so even after admitting that toxic mercury vapor is released from these fillings. Mercury is a poison and it's unequivocally hazardous to your health!

I've saved the discussion about the ADA's role in perpetuating the use of amalgam fillings for the end of this book. I did so because I wanted you to first hear the "other" side of the story about the toxicity of these fillings. It's now time to offer my opinon on the role the ADA has played, including its attempts to discourage mercury safe dentists from educating their patients about the health hazards of mercury fillings.

How the ADA Stifles Freedom of Speech

The method the ADA used to stifle the freedom of speech of mercury safe dentists was to add an Advisory Opinion (Section 5.A) to its Code of Professional Conduct in 1986, just two years after admitting mercury vapor is released from amalgam fillings. It reads as follows: *"Based on available scientific data, the ADA has determined that the removal of amalgam restorations from the non-allergic patient for the alleged purpose of removing toxic substances from the body, when such treatment is performed solely at the recommendation or suggestion of the dentist, is improper and unethical."* Even if the ADA based its conclusion on all of the scientific data available, that was 22 years ago! Thankfully, there are dentists, scientists, health professionals, and researchers who have been willing to keep up to date with the latest research on this subject.

Let's assume, for example, that a dentist has extensively researched the latest scientific literature and concluded that mercury is a poison, is released from amalgam fillings as a vapor, enters the body, and accumulates there. Based on this information, a dentist has no other choice but to inform his or her patients that amalgam fillings are a health hazard. Then, after evaluating the information provided by the dentist, the patient authorizes the dentist to safely remove his or her amalgam fillings and replace them with much safer fillings. To me, this course of action represents morally responsible and ethical dentistry. Given the fact that patients pay dentists to impart their knowledge and skills, I would expect no less. In fact, if I discovered my dentist withheld critically important information that could negatively affect my overall health (and more importantly, the health of my children), I wouldn't just be concerned, I'd be very upset.

So what could possibly be so wrong about a dentist telling a patient that amalgam fillings continuously emit a powerful poison? First, the ADA still considers amalgams to be a perfectly safe and harmless filling, even though it has admitted that amalgams release mercury vapor. As far as the ADA is concerned, if a dentist supposedly "talks" his or her patient into replacing amalgam fillings because the dentist says they are a health hazard, he or she is doing so to make a profit.

Doing so, according to the ADA's logic, is an ethics violation, and the ADA believes it is protecting you from greedy and unscrupulous dentists.

But the ADA's logic is seriously flawed. The real reason for replacing a toxic mercury-emitting filling has nothing to do with whether or not it's deemed a functional filling. It's about the fact that amalgam fillings are vehicles for delivering poisonous mercury vapor to the body. The dentists who should be sanctioned by the ADA are the ones who *don't* tell their patients that amalgam fillings release a powerful poison, not dentists who educate their patients about the health hazards of these fillings. Even so, the ADA has no problem with pro-amalgam dentists encouraging patients to replace amalgam fillings with a composite, purely for aesthetic/cosmetic reasons, while making a profit in the process. Logical? Fair? I think not! Hypocritical? I think so!

Through legislative lobbying, pro-amalgam media propaganda, avoiding the large body of scientific research, and exerting undue influence over state and local dental boards and dental schools, the ADA continues to support the safety of amalgam fillings and discourage those who disagree. The ADA is a very powerful organization and it has been very effective in silencing dentists who feel obligated to provide this information to their patients.

There's more. An article by Dr. Ilona Visser in *Natural Medicine* (Feb/March 2006) will help you understand how the ADA discourages anti-amalgam dentists from educating their patients about this subject by utilizing its power to revoke a dentist's license to practice. The article points out that over 40 dentists have been de-licensed by the state dental boards because of their stance against mercury fillings. It takes great courage to stand up to this powerful organization, especially given the fact that by doing so you could lose your livelihood.

What's Going on Here?

For the ADA to interfere with a dentist's right to inform his or her patients about their exposure to a toxic substance not only censures the dentist's right of free speech, but would be analogous to the American Medical Association (AMA) telling its doctors not to inform their patients about the health hazards of smoking. In spite of an overwhelming amount of scientific evidence to the contrary, the ADA continues to discourage dentists from telling their patients that:

- Their health is at risk from mercury fillings.

- They should consider having these fillings safely removed and replaced.

- They should see a qualified health professional to be tested for mercury poisoning.

- They should consider participating in a mercury detoxification program to remove the mercury that has accumulated in their bodies.

But why would the ADA *not* want dentists to educate their patients about *any* dental-related subject that could affect the patient's oral and overall health? I suggest that if it didn't attempt to discourage dentists from discussing the health hazards of amalgam fillings, it would, in effect, be admitting that amalgam fillings are a health hazard. Of course, the real question here is: "Whose health is being put at risk because of the ADA's efforts to hinder dentists from speaking the truth to their patients?"

Most dental patients are not aware of what is being put into their teeth, as a poll conducted by Zogby International (January 2006) reveals:

- 76 percent of respondents did not know mercury is the primary component of amalgam (silver) fillings.

- *92 percent wanted to be informed of their choices with respect to mercury and non-mercury dental filling materials prior to dental treatment.*

- 77 percent would choose higher-cost fillings that do not contain mercury if given the choice.

- 47 percent think mercury pollution poses a serious problem for the environment.

- 69 percent would support a ban on mercury amalgam fillings for children and pregnant women.

The ADA's Position and My Response

The ADA's approach has been to promote only one side of the amalgam story and encourage pro-amalgam dentists to tell their patients that amalgams are safe and harmless. I've been told that some pro-amalgam dentists still tell their patients that mercury *is not released from amalgam fillings*, even though the ADA has admitted that it is! Pro-amalgam dentists have a powerful voice because the ADA is speaking for them. To ensure this discussion is balanced, I'll be the advocate for mercury safe dentists. The following are what I understand to be the ADA's reasons for saying that mercury fillings are safe and harmless. I'll follow each statement with my response. (The ADA's position, as I interpret it, is italicized in quotations.)

"There are no studies that prove that amalgam fillings are a health hazard."

It's actually true that the amalgam filling itself isn't a health hazard, it's the mercury vapor released from it that creates the health problems. Thousands of studies have proven that mercury is a powerful poison and hundreds of studies have proven that amalgam fillings release toxic mercury vapor. Amalgam fillings are a health hazard because they are the vehicle that delivers mercury to the body! The ADA uses semantics to confuse the issue.

The ADA has never done a credible study proving that these fillings are safe. In fact, *no study exists* that has proven mercury fillings are, have ever been, or could ever be, safe. What's more, if, for the first time ever, the materials in amalgams were submitted to the FDA today for approval as a dental filling, it would never allow their use.

I've extensively researched this subject and have compiled nearly 1,100 scientific studies that deal with amalgam fillings, chronic mercury poisoning, and mercury detoxification. The references include an extensive table of contents, each article has been abstracted, and the majority of them contain a Pub Med reference number. I've included nearly 300 of them in the Reference section of this book.

"Amalgam is the best filling material for the price, and there's nothing better to replace it."

Years ago this may have been true, but it's far from true today. I wrote about composites and other replacement fillings in Chapter 9, and there is absolutely no doubt that the newest generations of composites are better than mercury fillings. In fact, in 2007, for the first time ever, more than 50 percent of dentists in the U.S. have said that they no longer use amalgam fillings because they know amalgam is not a good filling material and that better choices are available. In 2008, Denmark, Norway, and Sweden banned amalgams because of the effects of mercury on the environment and because better filling materials are available.

"If amalgam fillings were a health hazard, then after all these years of use, the dental profession would see evidence of it."

The ADA's claim that dentists don't see people with symptoms or illnesses related to mercury toxicity is blatantly false. Every day pro-amalgam dentists see patients who have a multitude of health problems, all of which could be contributed to, or worsened by, chronic exposure to mercury. I'm sure you remember filling out a health history form at the dental office that asks you to check an assortment of diseases and illnesses that you are experiencing. As you've read in this book, chronic mercury poisoning is connected to some extent, directly or indirectly, to every symptom or disease listed on that form.

You should know that the dentist doesn't request this health history information in order to treat you for the medical conditions you checked off, but to see if any of them, such as an allergy to penicillin or a heart condition, would affect your dental treatment. If the dentist looking at your medical history understood that chronic mercury poisoning affects every condition listed in the health history form, he or she would understand that the majority of patients with amalgam fillings will have a health issue directly or indirectly related chronic mercury poisoning. What I find to be hypocritical is that although the ADA acknowledges that a small percentage of people are allergic to mercury, it doesn't require dentists to ask that question of their patients.

"Dentists have been using amalgam fillings for over 150 years, and that proves they're safe."

The ADA's primary defense of amalgam fillings is based on the fact that amalgams have been used for over 150 years. In fact, absolutely no scientific evidence proves that the amount of time something has been in use has anything to do with its safety. The tobacco and asbestos industries said basically the same thing about their products. So did the paint industry when it put mercury and lead into its products. The truth is that if a toxic material has been used for a long time, that doesn't make it less toxic.

"The amount of mercury that amalgam fillings release is in such small quantities that it doesn't pose a health hazard."

I've extensively discussed this subject in the book but, as a refresher, *mercury is a powerful poison and there's no such thing as a safe level.* That means *any* amount entering the body poses a health hazard. The ADA might want you to believe that small amounts of mercury are safe, but Chapter 3 proves that what the ADA says about this simply isn't true.

"Even if small amounts of mercury enter the body daily, the body will be able to remove it and thus none will accumulate."

Absolutely not true! What is true is that the body has the ability to remove mercury. But as you know, over time its ability to remove mercury decreases, and more and more mercury will accumulate. According to the ADA, it's mercury in and mercury out. This theory makes the erroneous assumption that the body will be able to remove any amount of mercury that enters it. This might sound good to the ADA, but it has no factual basis.

If you took a fecal metals test for mercury prior to having your fillings removed, the test would show that mercury was indeed being removed by the body. But according to the ADA's mercury in and mercury out theory, if the fecal test was taken shortly after all amalgam fillings were removed, the test would show mercury levels equal to those who never had amalgam fillings.

But this isn't the case. You could do a fecal metals test every day for a year after amalgam removal and *each time* it would show higher levels of mercury than for those who never had an amalgam filling. This proves that the amount of mercury entering the body every day from amalgam fillings is not being removed every day. The ADA suggests that if testing still indicates high levels of mercury after filling removal, then the mercury must have come from contaminated fish. But that theory doesn't hold up either, because the mercury levels are still higher from those who had amalgams but who never consumed contaminated fish.

Protecting Your Mercury Safe Dentist

The best way to protect a mercury safe dentist is to specifically ask him or her to tell you what they know about mercury fillings. As I've explained, many mercury safe dentists are hesitant to initiate the discussion about the health hazards of amalgams. However, if *you* ask the dentist about these fillings it means *he or she* didn't initiate the conversation and can't be seen as trying to talk you into anything. The dentist is simply answering your questions to the best of his or her ability.

The second way to protect the mercury safe dentist is to enlist the support of your health practitioner. If a health professional recommends that a patient remove his or her mercury fillings, the ADA regards that recommendation as a legitimate reason for the dentist to do so. Understand that the health professional isn't suggesting the patient have amalgam fillings removed because they aren't structurally sound—it's because he or she knows amalgams are a source of highly poisonous mercury. As much as it disappoints the ADA, it hasn't been able to censure a dentist, or put him or her on probation, or revoke his or her license, for following the advice of a patient's physician or qualified health practitioner.

When asked why it continues to stifle anti-mercury dentists' freedom of speech, ADA officials have said that it's just trying to protect the public from "quacks" who falsely say mercury fillings are a health hazard. Based on the fact that 15 percent or more of dentists in the U.S. are mercury safe, and more than 50 percent no longer use amalgam, there must be a lot of "quacks" practicing dentistry! Astonishingly, and in spite of abundant evidence to the contrary, the ADA adamantly refuses to change its position. The good news is that it can't prevent a patient from asking questions, nor can it restrict dentists from providing information—*as long the patient has requested it.*

Testing for Mercury and the ADA's Response

The ADA doesn't recognize legitimate testing for mercury. It doesn't matter that the medical profession relies on such tests from licensed laboratories, and considers them to be proper diagnostic tools for heavy metal toxicity. A qualified health professional can say, based on test results, that the mercury released from amalgam fillings will directly or indirectly contribute to a patient's health issues. Amazingly, the ADA discourages dentists from saying the same thing, even though both base their opinions on the same tests.

One can only hope that as more and more information becomes available to health practitioners, they will understand that if a patient has amalgam fillings, each health issue is related to the mercury released from amalgam fillings to some degree. Once they cease to believe the ADA's stance on amalgams and objectively look at the solid evidence, I would hope these guardians of our health will recommend that *every* patient have his or her amalgam fillings safely removed.

Legal Implications

One of the most compelling factors that could affect the future of amalgam fillings in the U.S. is the lawsuit. The bulk of the scientific evidence connecting mercury vapor released from amalgam fillings to health problems began emerging in the 1980s and has increased exponentially since then. The time is rapidly approaching when the ADA will no longer be able to support its position regarding the safety of mercury fillings. It may still be able to exert great influence on member dentists, but it won't be able to stop patients from suing pro-amalgam dentists. Nor will the ADA be able to stop governmental agencies from restricting amalgams or the federal government from passing legislation banning these toxic fillings.

As the evidence increases, pro-amalgam dentists, the ADA, and its state and local affiliates are under more and more pressure to defend their "mercury fillings are safe for everyone" position. More and more individuals and organizations throughout the U.S. are filing lawsuits against the ADA, state and local dental associations, and pro-amalgam dentists. At the time of publication, none of these suits has been resolved, but the trend is clear. *The public is getting the message, they're angry, and they are fighting back!* These actions are encouraging. Awareness that mercury fillings are hazardous to human health is also filtering out to the media and finding its way into the legislative and legal system.

ADA Abandons Pro-Amalgam Dentists

The ADA might publicly act like it's fervently guarding its amalgam sand castle, but behind the scenes they're undoubtedly becoming more and more nervous about the anti-amalgam groundswell. In 1992, an attorney for the ADA filed a brief in the Superior Court of the State of California disassociating the ADA from liability for any health problem that could result from placing mercury amalgam fillings.

In its brief, the ADA stated that it has no legal duty to protect the public from allegedly dangerous products that dentists use. The ADA further stated that it doesn't manufacture, design, supply, mix, or place mercury-containing amalgams, and has no control over those who do. Hidden under the legalese is that the ADA won't protect pro-amalgam dentists from any legal backlash. In short, the ADA says it's not responsible for what the individual dentist does or doesn't do. Although I doubt the majority of ADA member pro-amalgam dentists know this, the ADA has effectively abandoned them on this key legal issue.

Furthermore, the ADA sought additional protection from future lawsuits by saying that just because it provides dentists with information about various products, this doesn't imply it has a duty to protect the patient from any injury resulting from the use of those products.

What It Means

What does the ADA's legal stance really mean? To me, it demonstrates a disregard for every dentist who has believed what the ADA told him or her about the safety of amalgams. More importantly, it demonstrates the ADA's hypocrisy by telling the public and its pro-amalgam supporters that amalgams are safe, while doing its best to stifle anti-amalgam dentists and disavow any legal liability for mercury amalgam fillings.

I firmly believe that if the ADA doesn't act responsibly and quickly to implement a ban on mercury fillings, lawyers or government regulation will take over. Dentistry can't afford to deal with class action lawsuits that would, in effect, shut down pro-amalgam dentists. Clearly, the writing is on the wall and the ADA should be reading it. It's time for the ADA to do the right thing and take the steps necessary to ban these poisonous fillings.

On a Positive Note

While I will remain a vocal critic of the ADA's position on mercury amalgam fillings until they are forever banned, the ADA does provide a valuable service to the dental community in many other areas, such as overseeing dental schools and certifying oral care products. It's too bad it has taken this archaic position on amalgams, and I believe this explains the ADA's dramatic decline in membership over the years. In fact, today 50 percent of dentists under 35 are not ADA members.

Changing the Law

A number of mercury free dental organizations, such as the International Association of Mercury Free Dentists (IAMFD), the International Academy of Oral Medicine and Toxicology (IAOMT), the International Academy of Biological Dentists and Medicine (IABDM), the Holistic Dental Association (HAD), Dental Amalgam Mercury Solutions (DAMS), thousands of supportive mercury safe dentists, and countless concerned private citizens are making positive inroads towards getting amalgam fillings banned by the FDA and other legislative bodies.

One of the staunchest advocates for having amalgams banned is Charles G. Brown, National Counsel for Consumers for Dental Choice. At present, he's leading the fight to have the FDA re-evaluate its position on these fillings and the FDA is now considering reclassifying amalgam. This effort has caught the ADA's attention. On July 1, 2007, in an update to its members regarding the FDA's possible actions on amalgams, the ADA sent the following information to its members (these are excerpts): "We don't know the direction the FDA will take; The FDA could issue a mandatory brochure or even limited warnings; The FDA could even issue 'a ban,' though we don't expect the latter."

Clearly the ADA is expressing some concern about its ability to defend the indefensible. If you'd like to add your name to those supporting the banning of these toxic fillings, go to my website, www.dentalwellness4u.com, and click on "Ban Mercury Amalgam Silver Fillings" in the Frequently Asked Questions (FAQ) menu. Your name will be included with other like-minded people and will be submitted to the appropriate legislator and government agency. I'll keep you updated on my website about the efforts being made via legal and legislative action.

Message for Pro-Amalgam Dentists

On the one hand, the ADA has repeatedly told you that amalgam is a perfectly safe and harmless filling material. On the other hand, it has abandoned you if you get sued for *not* informing your patients that amalgams release poisonous mercury vapor and are a health hazard. In a court of law it will be you, and you alone, who'll be held responsible for your actions, or inactions in this case, and I suggest that you seriously consider the ramifications.

I strongly encourage you to consult with an attorney and ask if you can legally use the defense that the ADA told you mercury fillings were safe and, without undertaking your own research, believed what they said. Then, ask if you can use ignorance as an excuse for exposing your patients to poisonous mercury without their consent. As I understand it, ignorance is no excuse in the eyes of the law, and I doubt that any court or jury (most of whom will have, or had, mercury fillings in their teeth) will let you get away with saying you were simply following the ADA's position. As a pro-amalgam dentist, you are likely to face two legal issues. The first is that amalgam fillings are a health hazard and you didn't inform your patients of that fact. The second is that during the placement and removal of amalgams, you exposed your patients to enormous amounts of mercury, didn't tell them, and didn't protect them.

Losing such a lawsuit could be devastating. Consider the available evidence, ask the right questions, and take the right action for yourself and your patients. I don't believe the ADA will support you in the event of legal action and, if in doubt, I suggest you contact the ADA and ask its representative if it will be a witness for your defense.

Two things need to be considered. The first is that you shouldn't put mercury amalgam fillings in your patients' teeth. The second is how to best protect your patients, yourself, your staff, and the environment from unnecessary exposure to mercury at the office when these fillings are placed and removed. It's critically important that you understand that the latter is a totally separate issue from the health hazards mercury amalgams pose to people who have them in their teeth. You may still want to argue that the mercury coming off a patient's amalgam fillings isn't significant enough to be harmful, but from reading this book, you now know that an enormous amount of mercury vapor is released when amalgams fillings are put in, removed, or polished.

The evidence against the safety of these fillings is overwhelming and there is **no** evidence proving mercury fillings are safe for anyone. Amalgam fillings aren't even considered to be a good filling material anymore, and I suggest that you've nothing to gain by supporting what I believe is the indefensible position the ADA has taken on amalgam fillings.

Taking a mercury safe approach means telling your patients that you've assumed a moral, if not legal, responsibility to make sure your office is as mercury safe as possible. The benefits to you are substantial, from both a health and legal standpoint, and to your patients, from the standpoint of minimizing mercury exposure. If you no longer use amalgams, you should understand that it isn't enough to just be mercury free—*you must also be mercury safe!* (If you're interested in becoming mercury safe, I consult with dentists about how to make their offices mercury safe. You can contact me at 800-335-7755 for more information.)

Message for Female Pro-Amalgam Dentists

I want to particularly reach out to female pro-amalgam dentists, especially if you are now, or plan to be, a mother. I suggest that you take a very close look at the effects of mercury on the fetus, nursing baby, and child in Chapter 6. You not only owe it to yourself to be open-minded and objective, but you also owe it to your patients who are pregnant, plan to be, or are nursing their babies. If there's even an iota of doubt in your mind about the safety of amalgam fillings, I find it hard to understand how you could continue to expose your female patients to mercury vapor when there's a viable, cost-effective and safe alternative. I strongly encourage you to reassess the morality, and the potential legal implications to you and your practice, of continuing to place these toxic fillings .

Message for Mercury Safe Dentists

I stopped using mercury amalgam fillings in 1970 and publically came out against them in 1972 when I wrote my first book about oral health for the layperson, *The Tooth Trip*. I know the road you've traveled and how difficult it has been for you to stand up against the ADA, state and local dental associations, and pressure from your peers. I consider every mercury safe dentist to be a hero in the fight to ban toxic amalgam fillings. I acknowledge you and applaud your courage and willingness to commit to mercury safe dentistry and in doing so, to protect the health of your patients, yourself, your staff, and the environment.

Although I wrote this book for the dental patient, it was also written with the mercury safe dentist in mind. Providing this book to your patients is the most cost- and time-effective way of educating interested patients about this subject away from the dental office. The book will also help protect you legally because you'll have provided your patients with the information they need to make an informed choice about these toxic fillings—from a credible third-party source. *The Poison in Your Teeth* will provide you with a safe and effective way to get this information out to them.

Today, more and more people are becoming aware of the value and importance of finding mercury safe dentists to safely remove amalgam fillings. It's estimated that over 60 percent of those searching for mercury free dentists find them on the Internet. To help people find mercury free dentists, I founded the Mercury Free Dentist Internet Listing Service. Becoming a member offers many advantages, the most important of which is to provide you with a prominent Internet presence, making it easy for people searching the internet for a mercury safe dentist to find you. You can learn about the many benefits and advantages of membership on my website, www.dentalwellness4u.com, or by calling 800-335-7755.

Other Countries and Mercury Fillings

The ADA may have a lot of influence in the U.S., but other developed countries don't see eye to eye with it regarding mercury fillings. In January 2008, Norway and Sweden banned the use of mercury amalgams as a dental material, and Denmark banned amalgams in April 2008. Germany and Austria have banned the use of mercury amalgam fillings in pregnant women and children up to age 18, and complete bans are scheduled to be phased in. Switzerland has banned dental schools from teaching the use of amalgam fillings, essentially amounting to an eventual ban in that country.

A number of states and cities in the U.S. have also taken action. California requires a warning notice be placed in all dental offices that have a staff of 10 or more and place amalgam fillings. The notice states: "The people of the state of California have determined that the use of dental amalgam causes birth defects and other health problems." Notice that it says the people—not the dentists— of California because the pro-amalgam faction intensely fought having this warning issued, delaying its implementation for years. Minnesota is proposing a similar approach to the one taken by California. And the Philadelphia City Council has voted to require dentists to give patients an informative fact sheet before placing amalgams.

The Future of Mercury Amalgam Fillings

In spite of the ADA's support for amalgam fillings, more than 50 percent of general dentists today no longer use them. That doesn't necessarily mean these dentists are mercury safe or believe that amalgam is a health hazard—for most it means that they don't think it is a good filling material. Nevertheless, this is still very encouraging news because 35 years ago probably one percent of dentists were mercury free.

One survey showed that 80 percent of dentists would stop using amalgams and switch to another filling material if it were available and had all of the same qualities of an amalgam filling, but without the mercury. I think by qualities they mean that the other filling material would be as easy to put in and be as inexpensive as amalgams.

The bottom line is that more and more dentists are shunning amalgam because amalgam fillings are toxic and the latest version of composites is simply a much better filling material. Ultimately, fewer dentists are using amalgams today because of attrition—most of the stubbornly pro-amalgam dentists are older and not willing to commit the time and expense needed to upgrade their practices and provide the latest generation of composites to their patients. So the natural process of attrition (retirement or passing away) means that each year more of the staunchest pro-amalgam dentists are gone and more modern, open-minded, objective dentists are taking their place.

The ultimate irony here is that if amalgam fillings were introduced today and submitted to the FDA as a dental filling material, they would **never** be approved for use. In fact, they wouldn't be approved for any purpose. Of course, that raises the question of why the FDA still allows the use of amalgam. The only answer to that question that makes sense is that the ADA's powerful lobby, paid for by its members' dues, has influenced the governmental agencies to look the other way.

Some Final Comments

Despite the ADA's efforts, the future for amalgam fillings is bleak. We live in the twenty-first century, the science and technology of today is light years from where it was 150 years ago, and I believe it is irresponsible to use ancient science to defend its position. Even though the ADA has failed in its responsibility to support objective research about the health hazards of mercury amalgam fillings, other countries throughout the world have done so, providing a wealth of information for those willing to take the time to find it. Ironically, and in spite of its intense support of amalgam fillings, the ADA can't provide a scientifically acceptable study proving that these fillings are safe!

Thankfully, we are fortunate to have access to the Internet and the bottomless wealth of knowledge it makes available. This has been so important to the mercury safe and anti-mercury faction, because the ADA can no longer control access to information about this subject. Each year more and more information is available about the health hazards of mercury fillings. And each year more and more people participate in the effort to ban these fillings, and seek out mercury safe dentists to have these poisonous fillings safely removed.

For over 30 years I've been involved with the movement to ban these fillings. I've watched this movement grow from a few to many—and I know the tide has turned. The writing is not just on the wall, it is etched in the wall, and I've no doubt amalgam fillings will soon be a historical footnote.

I encourage you to lend your voice to those who have worked so hard to have these fillings banned. You can support this heroic effort by going to my website and selecting "Ban Mercury Amalgam Silver Fillings" in the Frequently Asked Questions (FAQ) section of the homepage.

Testing for Mercury

Testing for mercury is the only way to objectively determine if your body is eliminating higher than normal amounts of mercury, or if it can be detected in the body. But even testing has limitations. For example, no test can tell you where and how much mercury is in your body, how much is in your brain, or exactly how much damage it has done.

In this section I will give a brief overview of each commonly used test, including the fecal metals, blood, urine, hair, and porphyrin profile tests. You can find more detailed information about these tests at www.dentalwellness4u.com by clicking on "Testing for Mercury" in the Frequently Asked Questions (FAQ) menu on the homepage. The contact information for the testing laboratories I recommend can be found in Appendix D, and each has as an informative website. But keep in mind that you'll need a health practitioner or dentist to order any of these tests for you.

Fecal Metals Test

Ninety percent of the mercury eliminated by the body's *natural* detoxification/chelation process is by way of the liver/common bile duct/intestine/feces pathway. Thus, any objective testing for mercury should include the fecal metals test. I also highly recommend this test for patients, dentists, or health practitioners who are skeptical about whether or not mercury has accumulated in the body, or would like to monitor the progress of a detoxification program.

While it's possible to use the fecal metals test only for mercury, I recommend you ask to be tested for the full range of toxic metals. The body can also remove other toxic metals along with mercury, so it's a good idea to keep track of them too. Doing so will help your dentist or health practitioner monitor which ones are being removed and their rate of removal. The fecal metals test doesn't require a chelating drug, is noninvasive, and can be done at home. The test results are compared to those who have never had mercury amalgam fillings. I believe the fecal metals test, properly interpreted, provides the most useful information of all of the commonly available tests.

Unprovoked Urine Mercury Test

The unprovoked urine mercury test is a simple test for mercury that doesn't require a pharmaceutical chelating agent. Because less than 10 percent of the mercury the body removes passes through the kidneys and out through the urine, an unprovoked urine mercury test can be misleading. It can easily indicate a relatively "safe" reading when in fact the total body burden of mercury could actually be much higher. Used alone it could lead you to believe that you aren't that mercury toxic, when you actually are. While this test can indicate the amount of mercury the body removes via the kidneys, I don't recommend it for evaluating your body burden of mercury, determining how much mercury is being removed from your body, or for deciding whether or not to participate in a mercury detoxification program.

Urine Mercury Challenge Test

The urine mercury challenge is a provoked test and will show a far greater amount of mercury being removed from the kidneys than the unprovoked urine test—especially for those who still have amalgam fillings. With this test, DMPS or DMSA is used. These pharmaceutical chelators are most commonly used to capture and remove mercury and are much more aggressive at removing mercury than the body's natural chelators. Unlike the body's natural chelators, which remove mercury via the feces, pharmaceutical chelators remove the mercury they capture via the kidneys/urine pathway.

Ideally, the urine challenge test should be done more than once, with the first test used as a reference. You can then compare the results of future tests with the first one. It's also important to note that pharmaceutical chelators aren't selective—they'll remove other metals along with mercury. For example, DMPS has a greater affinity for other metals, including zinc and copper, than it does for mercury.

This test has its value, especially if combined with the fecal metals test. But it also has its limitations. The fact that it requires a pharmaceutical chelator makes it unsuitable for babies, young children, and those who may be allergic to the chelator.

Blood Mercury Test

While this test can indicate exposure to all three types of mercury (elemental, inorganic, and organic), it can be misleading because it only tests for mercury found in the blood at the time the blood was drawn. It cannot be used to determine the body's *burden* of mercury, where the mercury is stored, the damage it is doing, or the body's effectiveness at removing it.

The test can also be misinterpreted if taken by those with amalgam fillings. Mercury vapor passes quickly through the lungs and into and out of the bloodstream. Thus, any exposure to elemental mercury vapor from amalgam fillings shortly before testing can dramatically affect the test results. For example, if you stimulated your fillings by chewing gum shortly before blood is drawn, the test could indicate a high level of blood mercury. But if your fillings weren't stimulated for two hours before the blood sample was taken, it could show low levels of blood mercury. Thus, the same person taking the same blood test at two different times could show two completely different results.

Unless it's indicated for other reasons, the blood test can be extremely misleading in determining how much mercury is actually in your body, or how much it is removing. I believe that unless a fecal metals test is also done, and the results compared, this isn't a meaningful test for mercury exposure from amalgam fillings. For example, mercury levels in the blood could indicate relatively "safe" levels while the fecal metals test could indicate high, harmful levels.

Hair Analysis

Anywhere from 70 to 95 percent of the mercury found in a hair sample comes from organic mercury. The main source of organic mercury is from contaminated fish. So, if you have high mercury hair levels, the majority of it could be from fish and not from the elemental mercury released by amalgam fillings. Thus, you could still be exposed to high levels of elemental mercury and yet show low readings of mercury in the hair. Many believe that the hair analysis is a good test for evaluating the body's mineral levels and, interpreted correctly, it can be helpful for that purpose. However, using hair analysis to evaluate the body's burden of mercury can be misleading.

Urine Porphyrin Profile

The urine porphyrin profile is a non-invasive test that can detect recent exposure to mercury but does so in an indirect way. It detects substances that show up in the urine because the body is being exposed to mercury. However, it's not reflective of the mercury that is stored in the body or of the mercury that the body removes naturally. The test is based on the fact that mercury blocks certain enzymes that are involved in converting a protein called porphyrin into heme (essential for formation of hemoglobin). The result is that more porphyrin will be excreted in the urine than if mercury wasn't present.

Based on my research, I think this test is useful in evaluating an ongoing exposure to mercury, especially from amalgam fillings. However, because it can't determine the amount of mercury the body is removing naturally I think it would be even more valuable if done in conjunction with a fecal metals test—particularly for those who've already had their amalgam fillings removed. It would also be a valuable test for dentists and staff in helping to determine the extent of their current mercury exposure.

MELISA® Test

The MELISA® test (Memory Lymphocyte Immuno Stimulation Assay) measures hypersensitivity to numerous metals, including mercury, by placing a series of metals into contact with the white blood cells of the person being tested and then evaluating the reaction to each. At the time of publication, this allergy test was the only scientifically proven test of this type.

Test results will enable you to confirm or eliminate the possibility that you're allergic to mercury or other heavy metals. This test would be useful if you have mercury fillings and also have allergies that haven't been accurately diagnosed, or if you haven't adequately responded to treatment for a suspected allergy. To avoid confusing a mercury allergy with an allergic reaction to another substance, I highly recommend the MELISA® test.

Subjective Evaluation

To my knowledge, there is no method of objectively determining the degree of an individual's exposure to mercury. But after years of researching this subject, I developed a simple Mercury Risk Evaluation which consists of three risk categories—low, moderate, and high—and is based on your own subjective self-evaluation. This subjective risk evaluation primarily focuses on your exposure to mercury from your amalgam fillings. But the evaluation also takes into consideration your general health and other sources of mercury exposure.

I recommend that you take this evaluation if you're concerned about mercury poisoning, even if you haven't yet experienced any symptoms related to chronic mercury poisoning. It will give you an indication as to where you are now—and the direction in which you're heading. Access the "Mercury Risk Evaluation" from the Frequently Asked Questions (FAQ) menu at www.dentalwellness4u.com

Other Sources of Mercury Exposure

Manufacturing

At the time of publication, there were over 3,000 industrial uses for mercury and its various compounds. That means that both the people who make these products and those who use them are at risk of mercury exposure. Fortunately, mercury is gradually being eliminated from many personal use products in the U.S. But if you work in the manufacturing of these products or use any of them, I suggest you check with the appropriate department to determine your risk of exposure. If you're not sure, write to the manufacturer and ask if that product still contains mercury.

The following table includes a list of the more common industrial uses of mercury.

Industrial Uses of Mercury	
Acetaldehyde Production	Fur Hat Processing
Antiseptics	Germicidal Agents
Antisyphilitic Agents	Gold Mining
Arc Lamps	Histology Products
Bactericide	Ink Manufacturing
Barometers	Infrared Detectors
Batteries	Insecticidal Products
Bronzing	Manometers
Calibration Instruments	Mercury Amalgam Fillings
Chemical Laboratories	Mirror Silvering

Industrial Uses of Mercury	
Chlor-Alki Production	Neon Lamps
Computers and CRTs	Paints
Cosmetics	Paper Pulp Products
Dental Offices	Pathology Products
Diaper Products	Perfumes
Electric Switches	Photography
Electroplating	Polyurethane Foam Production
Embalming Agents	Seed Preservation
Explosives	Semiconductor Cells
Fabric Softeners	Silver and Gold Production
Farming Industry	Spermicidal Jellies
Finger Printing Products	Tattooing Inks
Floor Waxes and Polishes	Taxidermy Production
Fluorescent and Mercury Lamps	Thermometers
Fossil Fuel Production	Vaccine Preservatives
Fungicide Products	Wood Preservatives

Environmental Sources

Environmental sources of mercury refers to exposure to mercury in the environment, such as from metal processing, incineration of fossil fuels (coal/oil/gas) and medical waste, the cremation process, and gold mining. Most of the mercury from these sources will find its way into the soil, water and air. The present world production of mercury is about 18,000,000 lbs (8,181,818 kg) per year. In 1994, electricity generated by burning fossil fuels was responsible for 23 percent of all mercury emissions, with coal-fired power plants emitting the most mercury. Living downwind from any facility that releases mercury will expose you to airborne mercury. The surrounding area will also have greater soil, river, lake, and groundwater contamination. Mercury released into the environment from dental offices is also a significant source of environmental contamination.

Dietary Exposure to Mercury

Sadly, we now know that a number of larger ocean fish have been contaminated with high levels of toxic organic mercury. The exposure takes place when elemental mercury enters the water from polluters such as coal-fired power plants, gold mining and accidental mercury release from companies using mercury in their products. Microorganisms absorb this elemental mercury, convert it to organic mercury, and then it's passed up the food chain to the larger fish. The reason larger fish are the most toxic is that they have a much longer time to accumulate mercury. Just 6 ounces (170 grams) of contaminated fish can contain the following amounts of mercury:

- Swordfish and shark—170 mcg

- Larger species of tuna, such as bluefin and yellow tail—68 mcg

- Smaller species of tuna, such as Albacore—35 mcg

Compare this to the Environmental Protection Agency's (EPA) maximum of 38.5 mcg of mercury intake *per week* for a person weighing 120 lbs (55.5 kg). I am disappointed that such an influential organization as the EPA can state that it's safe to consume 38.5 mcg of mercury in a week when *not one microgram of mercury is safe*. If the EPA took into consideration an individual's total intake of mercury, *from all sources*, it would need to reevaluate its position.

Fish to Avoid

In fact, this source of mercury contamination is so widespread that the Food and Drug Administration (FDA) now recommends that children, pregnant and nursing women, and all women of childbearing age should not consume *any* of the following fish species:

Fish to Avoid	
Swordfish	Grouper
Sea Bass	Orange Roughy
Halibut	Marlin
Tuna	Tile Fish
Shark	King Mackerel

Due to the amount of mercury found in these fish, I recommend that *everyone* who has or had amalgam fillings should avoid eating mercury-contaminated fish until their mercury levels have decreased significantly and mercury-related symptoms have been eliminated. Although the fish listed above are excellent sources of omega 3 fatty acids, you do have other options. There are fish species that haven't been contaminated with mercury, and you can also use mercury-free supplements to supply omega 3 to your diet.

To protect itself, the FDA also recommends that no one eat more than 12 ounces per week of the fish listed as *safe*. (A typical serving size of fish is from three to six ounces.) In addition, the EPA recommends that those in the mercury sensitive group—children and pregnant women—restrict fish consumption to one meal per week. To calculate the amount of mercury you'll receive from over 75 types of seafood and freshwater fish, visit www.gotmercury.org. This useful website will also calculate the amount you'd receive per serving and will compare it to the amount the EPA considers safe.

Even though all fresh and saltwater fish and shellfish will have some mercury, shellfish and smaller fresh and saltwater fish are generally considered safe. These include:

Safe Fresh and Saltwater Fish and Seafood	
Sardines	Sole
Tilapia	Salmon
Bass	Trout
Catfish	Crab
Cod	Crawfish
Oysters	Plaice

Something to Think About

The worst case scenario is that you could be exposed to mercury from your fillings, your workplace, the environment, products that you use, *and* your diet. You might not be able to control every source of exposure, but you can do a great deal by eliminating amalgam fillings and avoiding mercury-contaminated fish.

The Relationship of Oral Health to Overall Health

Although this book is about mercury fillings, that isn't the only oral health issue that can have a damaging effect on your overall health. You must take into account a number of other oral health concerns if you want to feel better, have more energy, live longer, and enjoy life to the fullest. In regards to their negative impact on your overall health, the most important of these "other" oral issues are:

- periodontal (gum) disease

- infected root canals

- jaw infections (also referred to as cavitations)

- allergy to dental materials

- fluoride

No matter what else you do to improve your overall health—including removing your mercury fillings—it's important to understand how your oral health affects your overall health. Most people are unaware that oral health issues can harm overall health. Yet if *all* of the oral health problems aren't acknowledged as being significant obstacles to attaining optimal health, any effort you undertake to treat existing health problems will simply not achieve the desired results. The fact is, you can't be healthy without good oral health.

Take gum disease as an example. The scientific evidence clearly demonstrates the harmful role it plays in serious and even life-threatening diseases. Gum disease can:

- increase the risk of heart attack by as much as 25 percent

- increase the risk of stroke by a factor of 10

- increase the severity of diabetes

- contribute to low preterm birth weights

- contribute to respiratory disease

- contribute to osteoporosis

- interfere with proper digestion

- severely stress the immune system

- dramatically lower resistance to other infections

Connecting the Dots

It's not difficult to connect the dots here—gum disease can contribute to all kinds of health issues. And once you make that connection, it's easy to appreciate how oral health problems can actually shorten your life expectancy. If you're committed to improving your overall health, you must be willing to make a commitment to eliminating *all* forms of dental disease, not just removing mercury fillings.

Space doesn't allow me to discuss all of the oral health issues that can affect your overall health, but I recommend that you talk to your physician or alternative health practitioner about including the status of your oral health when diagnosing your medical problems. You can get more information about the important relationship of oral to overall health from the Dental Wellness Institute (www.dentalwellness4u.com). I founded the Dental Wellness Institute in 1997 with the goal of educating the public about dental wellness and bridging the gap between the dental and medical professions. The website offers over 170 pages of information on every aspect of oral health, including links and other resources to support your efforts.

You can also access information about my latest books on oral health, how to eliminate gum disease and tooth decay, improve your oral and overall health, increase your life-expectancy, avoid or minimize costly gum surgery, save thousands of dollars in dental treatment costs, improve your immune system, and increase your energy.

Appendix D

Resources

The following list provides information about a number of holistic dental organizations, testing laboratories, and products I recommend. I have a high regard for all of them. In addition, www.dentalwellness4u.com has extensive "Resources" and "Links" sections.

Associations and Organizations

International Association of Mercury Free Dentists (IAMFD)
www.dentalwellness4u.com
This association provides a prominent Internet presence for dentists committed to mercury safe dentistry. The IAMFD's Mercury Free Dentist Internet Listing Service has one of the largest listings of mercury safe dentists in the world and its purpose is to help dentists and patients find each other. For patients, the listing includes extensive information about member dentists for easy evaluation. Today, over 60 percent of the people searching for mercury safe dentists find them on the Internet, and this listing service provides dentists with the prominent Internet presence needed to bring new patients to their practice. If you are a mercury safe dentist and want more information about the benefits of this listing service for you, your practice, and your patients, please call me toll free at 800-335-7755.

The International Academy of Oral Medicine and Toxicology (IAOMT)

The IAOMT is a science-based membership organization for dental, medical, and research professionals who seek to promote medical-dental cooperation, mercury free and mercury safe dentistry, and elevate standards of biocompatibility to products and materials used in the dental practice. I recommend this science-based organization to any dentist who wants to become mercury safe. It's a great organization to belong to if you're a mercury safe dentist. www.iaomt.org

The International Academy of Biological Dentistry and Medicine (IABDM)

The IABDM is an organization of physicians and holistic dentists who practice the art and science of biological dentistry. They research alternative treatments and materials that can be incorporated into the dental practice to help improve the oral and overall health of their patients. I recommend this organization for any dentist who wants to expand his or her dental knowledge beyond what was taught in dental school. www.iabdm.org

Holistic Dental Association (HDA)

The HDA was formed by a group of dentists who wanted a forum for the development and sharing of health-promoting therapies. This association provides information and guidance to those seeking to participate in their own health care and helps in the continuing education of dental and health practitioners who want to expand their knowledge and awareness. www.holisticdental.org

The Institute of Nutritional Dentistry (IND)

The IND is a unique teaching organization. It offers seminars specifically designed to teach dentists how to effectively practice whole body and healthy dentistry. The seminars provide dentists with access to the latest information on all aspects of nutritional dentistry, including innovative technology, products, and biocompatible dental materials. www.naturaldentistry.org

Dental Amalgam Mercury Solutions (DAMS)

DAMS is a patient support group providing information to mercury toxic individuals on testing and treatment options, which also features a list of specially trained dentists and doctors. It has provided information to many thousands of mercury-poisoned people, most of whose health improves significantly with proper treatment after reducing mercury exposure. DAMS is an excellent source of information about the toxicity of mercury amalgam fillings. www.amalgam.org

Dental Wellness Institute (DWI)
The Institute was founded by Tom McGuire, DDS, to bridge the gap between oral and overall health and to educate the public, dentists, and health professionals about the importance of oral health. A leading authority on oral health and chronic mercury poisoning, he has written a number of popular and informative books on preventive dentistry and mercury amalgam fillings for the layperson, including *The Poison in Your Teeth*, *Mercury Detoxification: The Natural Way to Remove Mercury from Your Body*, *Tooth Fitness: Your Guide to Healthy Teeth*, and *The Tooth Trip*. Dr. Tom offers office and phone consultations on prevention, impartial second opinions on dental treatment, and mercury detoxification. For more information about Dr. Tom, and to order his books, preventive dental products, and mercury detoxification supplements, please visit his website: www. dental wellness4u.com. Phone: 800-335-7755. Email: dentwell@pacbell.net.

Testing Laboratories

There are a number of very good laboratories that test for mercury. While other dental and health professionals may choose different laboratories, I've worked with most of those listed below, and recommend them as excellent places to start. If you want more information, call, email, or visit their websites.

Fecal Metals Test, Hair Analysis, Urine Challenge, and Blood Tests
Doctors Data, Inc.
    3755 Illinois St.
    Charles, IL 60174-7860
    Phone: 630-377-8139
    Toll free: 800-323-2784
    Fax: 630-587-7860
    Email: inquiries@doctorsdata.com
    Website: www.doctorsdata.com

Urine Porphyrin Profile
Metametrix Clinical Laboratory
    3425 Corporate Way
    Duluth, GA 30096
    Phone: 770-446-5483
    Toll free: 800-221-4640
    Email: inquiries@metametrix.com
    Website: www.metametrix.com

Mercury Allergy Test (MELISA®)
MELISA® Diagnostics
   Phone: 800-650-7850
   Fax: 650-641-2184
   Email: lana@melisa.org
   Website: http://melisadiagnostics.com
   Additional information about the MELISA® Foundation can be found at www.melisa.org.

Dental Materials Biocompatibility Test
Clifford Consulting and Research
   2275 J Waynoka Road
   Colorado Springs, CO 80915
   Phone: 719-550-0008
   Fax: 719-550-0009
   Website: www.ccrlab.com (Clifford Consulting has a very informative website, for both the layperson and the health professional.)

Testing for Glutathione
Mercury depletes glutathione (GSH), so your health practitioner may want to have you tested for GSH levels. An effective and relatively inexpensive method of indicating the body's GSH levels is to test for it in red blood cells. Immunosciences Lab (www.immuno-sci-lab.com) offers this test.

   Great Smokies Diagnostic Lab (GSDL) offers an assessment of the glutathione detoxification pathway in its Comprehensive Detox panel. GSDL is now Genova Diagnostics and can be accessed on the Internet by going to www.gdx.net/home.

   An analysis of urinary organic acids will also give an indirect assessment of GSH status, particularly in the skeletal muscles and kidneys. This test is available at Great Plains Laboratory (www.greatplainslaboratory.com) and Metametrix Clinical Laboratory (www.metametrix.com).

   A measurement of glutathione function in lymphocytes is offered by SpectraCell Laboratories (www.spectracell.com).

Products

Arizona Instruments, LLC
Jerome Mercury Vapor Analyzer
   1912 West 4th Street,Tempe, AZ 85281

800-390-1414
www.azic.com
Contact: Brad Hays

Isolite Systems

Isolite Dry Field Illuminator
2060 Alameda Padre Serra, Suite #20
Santa Barbara, CA 93103
Phone: 805-560-9888
Toll Free: 800-560-6066
www.isolitesystems.com
info@isolitesystems.com

Appendix E
References

American Dental Association

ADA acknowledges mercury is released from amalgam fillings: www.ada.org/public/media/releases/0207_release01.asp

ADA Letter: John W. Stanford, PhD. Secretary CDMIE. May 22, 1986.

Amalgam OK during pregnancy, ADA News 36:18, 2005.

American Dental Association's Special Report: The ADA and CDA Principals of Ethics and Code of Professional Conduct ADA Resolution 42H-1986. Transaction 1986:536.

Code of Professional Conduct Section E: ADA's Special Report: The ADA Principals of Ethics. Journal of the American Dental Association (April, 1990).

JADA. NIDR Workshop Vol. 109 9/84.

Patents on amalgams by the ADA. U. S. Patent #4,018,600, April 19, 1977. U. S. Patent # 4,078,921, March 14, 1978. Both patents have since expired.

The Superior Court of the State of California, Santa Clara County. Case No. 718228, Demurrer (October 22, 1992).

When Your Patients Ask about Mercury in Amalgams. ADA Division of Scientific Affairs. JADA, 120-395-8, 1990.

Mercury from amalgam fillings versus other sources

World Health Organization: Environmental Health Criteria Series, 1991.

Antioxidants

General

Influence of amalgam fillings on Hg levels and total antioxidant activity in plasma of healthy donors. Pizzichini M, et al. Sci Total Environ. 2003 Jan 1; 301(1–3):43–50.

Glutathione

Neurodegenerative disorders in humans: the role of glutathione in oxidative stress-mediated neuronal death. Bains JS, et al. Brain Res Brain Res Rev. 1997 Dec; 25(3):335–58.

Cysteine metabolism and metal toxicity. Quig D. Altern Med Rev. 1998 Aug;3(4):262–7. Doctor's Data, Inc., West Chicago, IL, USA. dquig@doctorsdata.com.

Autism

Autism, an extreme challenge to integrative medicine. Part 2: medical management. Kidd PM. Altern Med Rev. 2002 Dec; 7(6):472–99.

Autism: a novel form of mercury poisoning. Bernard S, et al. Med Hypotheses. 2001 Apr; 56(4):462–71.

Reduced levels of mercury in first baby haircuts of autistic children. Holmes AS, Blaxill MF, Haley BE. Int J Toxicol. 2003 Jul–Aug; 22(4):277–85.

The role of mercury in the pathogenesis of autism. Bernard S., et al. Mol Psychiatry 2002;7 (Suppl 2):S42–S43.

Bleaching

Effect of home bleaching products on mercury release from an admixed amalgam. Robertello FJ, et al. Am J Dent. 1999 Oct; 12(5):227–30.

Blood and body fluids

The contribution of dental amalgam to mercury in blood. Snapp KR, et al. J Dent Res. 1989 May; 68(5):780–5.

Metal exposure from amalgam alters the distribution of trace elements in blood cells and plasma. Lindh U., et al. Clin Chem Lab Med 2001;39:134–46–142.

Brain/CNS/Neurological

Application of a latent variable model for a multicenter study on early effects due to mercury exposure. Lucchini R, et al. Neurotoxicology. 2003 Aug; 24(4–5):605–16.

Chronic Elemental Mercury Intoxication: Neuropsychological Follow Up Case Study. Hua MS, et al. Brain Inj. 1996 May; 10(5):377–84.

Comparison of the developmental effects of two mercury compounds on glial cells and neurons in aggregate cultures of rat telencephalon. Monnet-Tschudi F, et al. Brain Res. 1996 Nov 25; 741(1–2):52–9.

Correlation of dental amalgam with mercury in brain tissue. Eggleston DW, et al. J Prosthet Dent. 1987 Dec; 58(6):704–7.

Defensive characteristics in individuals with amalgam illness as measured by the percept-genetic method Defense Mechanism Test. Henningsson M, et al. Acta Odontol Scand. 1996 Jun; 54(3):176–81.

Entry of low doses of mercury vapor into the nervous system. Pamphlett R, Coote P. Neurotoxicology. 1998 Feb; 19(1):39–47.

Improvement of Nerve and Immunological Damages after Amalgam Removal. Daunderer M. Amer. J. Of Probiotic Dentistry and Medicine, Jan 1991. www.rmdentalcentre.com/article.cfm?artid=4&catid=1.

Mercury neurotoxicity: mechanisms of blood-brain barrier transport. Aschner M, et al. Neurosci Biobehav Rev. 1990 Summer; 14(2):169–76.

Mercury vapor inhalation inhibits binding of GTP to tubulin in rat brain: Similarity to a molecular lesion in Alzheimer diseased brain. Pendergrass JC, et al. Neurotoxicology. 1997; 18(2):315–24.

Metals and free radicals in neurodegeneration. Olanow CW, et al. Curr Opin Neurol. 1994 Dec; 7(6):548–58.

Motor neuron uptake of low dose inorganic mercury. Pamphlett R., et al. J Neurol Sci 1996;135:63–67.

Neurobehavioral effects from exposure to dental amalgam Hg(o): new distinctions between recent exposure and Hg body burden. Echeverria D, et al. FASEB J. 1998 Aug;12(11):971–80.

Neurological and neurophysiological study of chloralkali workers previously exposed to mercury vapour. Andersen A, et al. Acta Neurol Scand. 1993 Dec; 88(6):427–33.

Neuropsychiatric sequelae of mercury poisoning. The Mad Hatter's disease revisited. O'Carroll RE, et al. Br J Psychiatry. 1995 Jul; 167(1):95–8.

Oxidative damage to nuclic acids in motor neurons containing mercury. Pamphlett R., et al. J Neurol Sci 1998;159:121–126.

Psychometric evidence that mercury from silver dental fillings may be an etiological factor in depression, excessive anger, and anxiety. Siblerud RL, et al. Psychol Rep. 1994 Feb; 74(1):67–80.

Shrinkage of Motor Axons Following Systemic Exposure to Inorganic Mercury. Pamphlett R, et al. J Neuropathol Exp Neurol. 1998 Apr; 57(4):360–6.

Silent latency periods in methylmercury poisoning and in neurodegenerative disease. Weiss B, et al. Environ Health Perspect. 2002 Oct; 110 Suppl 5:851–4.

Subjective symptoms and neurobehavioral performances of ex-mercury miners at an average of 18 years after the cessation of chronic exposure to mercury vapor. Mercury Workers Study Group. Kishi R, et al. Environ Res. 1993 Aug; 62(2):289–302.

Uptake of inorganic mercury by the human brain. Pamphlett R, et al. Acta Neuropathol (Berl). 1996 Nov; 92(5):525–7.

Breast milk

Exposure to toxic elements via breast milk. Oskarsson A, et al. Analyst. 1995 Mar; 120(3):765–70.

Mercury from maternal "silver" tooth fillings in sheep and human breast milk. A source of neonatal exposure. Vimy MJ, et al. Biol Trace Elem Res. 1997 Feb; 56(2):143–52.

The Mercury Concentration in Breast Milk Resulting from Amalgam Fillings and Dietary Habits. Drexler H, et al. Environmental Research, 1998;77(2):124–129.

Total and inorganic mercury in breast milk and blood in relation to fish consumption and amalgam fillings in lactating women. Oskarsson A, et al. Arch Environ Health 1996; 51:234–241. Arch Environ Health. 1996 May–Jun; 51(3):234–41.

Cellular damage

Ag, Cu, Hg, and Ni ions alter the metabolism of human monocytes during extended low-dose exposures. Wataha JC, et al. J Oral Rehabil. 2002 Feb; 29(2):133–9.

Comparison of the interaction of methyl mercury and mercuric chloride with murine macrophages. Christensen MM, et al. Arch Toxicol. 1993; 67(3):205–11.

Mercury-induced apoptosis in human lymphocytes: caspase activation is linked to redox status. Shenker BJ, et al. Antioxid Redox Signal. 2002 Jun; 4(3):379–89.

Mercury intolerance in relation to superoxide dismutase, glutathione peroxidase, catalase, and the nitroblue tetrazolium responses. Marcusson JA., et al. Environ Res 2000;83:123–128.

Methyl mercury, mercuric chloride, and silver lactate decrease superoxide anion formation and chemotaxis in human polymorphonuclear leucocytes. Obel N, et al. Hum Exp Toxicol. 1993 Sep; 12(5):361–4.

Oxidative mechanisms underlying methyl mercury neurotoxicity. Sarafian T, et al. Int J Dev Neurosci. 1991; 9(2):147–53.

Oxidative Metabolism of neutrophils in vitro and human mercury intolerance. Marcusson JA., et al. Toxicol In vitro 1998;12:383–388.

Role of glutathione metabolism in the glutamate-induced programmed cell death of neuronal-like PC12 cells. Froissard P, et al. Eur J Pharmacol. 1997 May 12; 326(1):93–9.

Studies on Hg (II)-induced H2O2 formation and oxidative stress in vivo and in vitro in rat kidney mitochondria. Lund BO, et al. Biochem Pharmacol. 1993 May 25; 45(10):2017–24.

Toxic metals and oxidative stress part I: mechanisms involved in metal-induced oxidative damage. Ercal N, et al. Curr Top Med Chem. 2001 Dec; 1(6):529–39.

Dentists and dental office

Behavioral effects of low-level exposure to elemental Hg among dentists. Echeverria D., et al. Neurotoxicol Teratol. 1995;17:161–168.

Behavioral effects of low-level exposure to Hgo among dental professionals: a cross-study evaluation of psychomotor effects. Bittner AC Jr., et al. Neurotoxicol Teratol. 1998;20:429–439.

Blood mercury levels of dental students and dentists at a dental school. Tezel H., et al. Br Dent J 2001;191:449–452.

Chronic low-level mercury exposure and neuropsychological functioning. Uzzell, B.P., et al. J of Clin and Exper Neuropsych. 8, 581–593. www.fasebj.org/cgi/content/full/12/11/971.

Chronic neurobehavioural effects of elemental mercury in dentists. Ngim CH, et al. Br J Ind Med. 1992 Nov; 49 (11):782–90.

Health and neuropsychological functioning of dentists exposed to mercury. Ritchie KA, et al. Occup Environ Med. 2002 May; 59(5):287–93.

Mercury and arsenic levels among Lebanese dentists: a call for action. Harakeh S., et al. Bull Environ Contam Toxicol 2003;70:629–635.

Mercury exposure of the population. IV. Mercury exposure of male dentists, female dentists and dental aides. Zander D, et al. Zentralbl Hyg Umweltmed. 1992 Dec; 193(4):318–28.

Neurobehavioral Effects from Exposure to Dental Amalgam Hgo: New Distinctions Between Recent Exposure and Hg Body Burden. Echeverria, et al., FASEB J. 12, 971–980 (1998).

Neuropsychological effects of low mercury exposure in dental staff in Erzurum, Turkey. Aydin N., et al. Int Dent J 2003;53:85–91.

Neurophysiological and neuropsychological function in mercury-exposed dentists. Shapiro, I.M., et al. The Lancet 1, 1147–1150 (1982).

Skeletal muscle abnormalities associated with occupational exposure to mercury vapours. Nadorfy-Lopez E., et al. Histol Histopathol 2000;15:673–682.

Sodium Dimercaptopropane-1-Sulfonate Challenge Test for Mercury in Humans: II. Urinary Mercury, Porphyrins and Neurobehavioral Changes of Dental Workers in Monterrey, Mexico. Gonzalez-Ramirez, D; et al. J Pharmocol Exper Therap, 272(1):264–74 (1995).

Suicide among Swedish dentists. A ten-year follow-up study. Arnetz BB, et al. Scand J Soc Med. 1987; 15(4):243–6.

Diseases and conditions

Alzheimer's

ADP-Ribosilation of Brain Neuronal Proteins is Altered by In Vitro and In Vivo Exposure to Inorganic Mercury. Palkiewicz, P.l., et al. Journal of Neurochemistry 62: 2049–2052, 1994.

Alzheimer Disease: Mercury as a Pathogenetic Factor and Apolipoprotein E as a Moderator. Mutter. Neuroendocrinol Letter. 2004; 25(5):275–283.

Hg2+ Induces GTP-Tubulin Interactions in Rat Brain Similar to Those Observed in Alzheimer's Disease. Haley, B., et al. Federation of American Societies for Experimental Biology (FASEB). 75th Annual Meeting. Atlanta, GA 21–25 April 1991. Abstract 493.

Amalgams and Alzheimer's disease (AD). Boyd Haley. www.whale.to/d/haley.html.

Imbalances of trace elements related to oxidative damage in Alzheimer's disease brain. Cornett CR, et al. Neurotoxicology. 1998 Jun; 19(3):339–45.

Increased blood mercury levels in patients with Alzheimer's disease. Hock C, et al. J Neural Transm. 1998; 105(1):59–68.

Mercury induced Alzheimer's disease: accelerating incidence? Ely JT. Bull Environ Contam Toxicol 2001;67:800–806.

Mercury induces cell cytotoxicity and oxidative stress and increases beta-amyloid secretion and tau phosphorylation in SHSY5Y neuroblastoma cells. Olivieri G, et al. J Neurochem. 2000 Jan; 74(1):231–6.

Mercury Vapor Inhalation Inhibits Binding of GTP to Tubulin in Rat Brain: Similarity to a Molecular Lesion in Alzheimer's Disease Brain. Pendergrass, J. C., et al., Neurotoxicology 18(2), 315–324 (1997).

Retrograde Degeneration of Neurite Membrane Structural Integrity of Nerve Growth Cones Following In Vitro Exposure to Mercury. Leong, CCW, et al., Neuroreport, vol.12, pps. 733–737 (2001).

The relationship of toxic effects of mercury to exacerbation of the medical condition classified as alzheimer's disease (2002). Haley B. www.fda.gov/ohrms/dockets/dailys/02/Sep02/091602/80027dd5.pdf.

Amyotrophic Lateral Sclerosis (ALS)

Amyotrophic lateral sclerosis after accidental injection of mercury. Schwarz S., et al. J Neurol Neurosurg Psychiatry 1996;60:698.

Amyotrophic lateral sclerosis and mercury—preliminary report. Mano Y, et al. Rinsho Shinkeigaku. 1990 Nov; 30(11):1275–7.

Effects of metals on the nervous system of humans and animals. Carpenter DO. Int J Occup Med Environ Health. 2001; 14(3):209–18.

Mercury intoxication simulating amyotrophic lateral sclerosis. Adams CR., et al. JAMA 1983;250:642–643.

Recovery from amyothrophic lateral sclerosis and from allergy after removal of dental amalgam fillings. Rehde O., et al. Int J Risk Safety Med 1994;4:229–236.

Arthritis

Mercury poisoning: an unusual cause of polyarthritis. Karatas GK, et al. Clin Rheumatol. 2002 Feb; 21(1):73–5.

Autoimmunity and Heavy Metals. Bigazzi PE. Lupus. 1994; 3: 449–453. Autoimmunity and heavy metals. Lupus. 1994 Dec; 3(6):449–53.

Cancer

Molecular mechanisms of metal toxicity and carcinogenesis. Wang S, et al. Mol Cell Biochem. 2001 Jun; 222(1–2):3–9.

Number of amalgam fillings in relation to cardiovascular disease, diabetes, cancer and early death in Swedish women. Ahlqwist M., et al. Community Dent Oral Epidemiol 1993;21:40–44.

Trace elements and thyroid cancer. Zaichick VYe, et al. Analyst. 1995 Mar; 120(3):817–21.

Candida

Candida albicans therapy. Is there ever an end to it? Dental mercury removal: an effective adjunct. Zamm AV. J. Orthomol. Med. 1, 1986, 261–266.

Chronic Fatigue Syndrome

Mercury and nickel allergy: risk factors in fatigue and autoimmunity. Sterzl I, et al. Neuroendocrinol Lett. 1999; 20(3–4):221–228.

Metal-specific lymphocytes: biomarkers of sensitivity in man. Stejskal VD, et al. Neuroendocrinol Lett. 1999; 20(5):289–298.

Reactions to metals in patients with chronic fatigue and autoimmune endocrinopathy. Sterzl I, et al. Vnitr Lek. 1999 Sep; 45(9):527–31.

The frequency of mercury intolerance in patients with chronic fatigue syndrome and healthy controls. Marcusson JA. Contact Dermatitis 1999;41:60–61.

Diabetes

Neurologic features of chronic minamata disease (organic mercury poisoning) and incidence of complications with aging. Uchino M, et al. J Environ Sci Health B. 1995 Sep; 30(5):699–715.

Number of amalgam fillings in relation to cardiovascular disease, diabetes, cancer and early death in Swedish women. Ahlqwist M., et al. Community Dent Oral Epidemiol 1993;21:40–44.

Fibromyalgia
Mercury exposure from dental amalgam fillings in the etiology of primary fibromyalgia: a pilot study. Kotter I, Durk H, Saal JG, Kroiher A, Schweinsberg F. J Rheumatol. 1995 Nov; 22(11):2194–5.

Hearing
Evidence that mercury from dental amalgam may cause hearing loss in multiple sclerosis patients. Siblerud RL, et al. Journal of Orthomolecular Medicine. 1997. Vol. 12. 240–44.

Heart
Effects of mercury on myosin ATPase in the ventricular myocardium of the rat. Moreira CM., et al. Comp Biochem Physiol C Toxicol Pharmacol 2003;135C:269–275.
Effects of small concentrations of mercury on the contractile activity of the rat ventricular myocardium. de Assis GP., et al. Comp Biochem Physiol C Toxicol Pharmacol 2003;134:375–383.
Intake of mercury from fish, lipid peroxidation, and the risk of myocardial infarction and coronary, cardiovascular, and any death in eastern Finnish men. Salonen JT, et al. Circulation. 1995 Feb 1; 91(3):645–55.
Mercury and idiopathic dilated cardiomyopathy. Lorscheider F., et al. J Am Coll Cardiol 2000;35:819–820.
Mortality from cardiovascular diseases and exposure to inorganic mercury. Boffetta P., et al. Occup Environ Med 2001;58:461–466.
Number of amalgam fillings in relation to cardiovascular disease, diabetes, cancer, and early death in Swedish women. Ahlqwist M., et al. Community Dent Oral Epidemiol 1993;21:40–44.
The relationship between mercury from dental amalgam and the cardiovascular system. Siblerud RL. Sci Total Environ. 1990 Dec 1; 99(1–2):23–35.

Herpes
Effect of mercuric chloride on macrophage-mediated resistance mechanisms against infection with herpes simplex virus type 2. Ellermann-Eriksen S, et al. Toxicology. 1994 Nov 11; 93(2–3):269–87.

Kidney
Mercury from dental "silver" tooth fillings impairs sheep kidney function, Boyd, N.D., et al. The American Physiological Society, 11: 1010–1014, 1991.
Mercuric ion attenuates nuclear factor-kappaB activation and DNA binding in normal rat kidney epithelial cells: implications for mercury-induced nephrotoxicity. Dieguez-Acuna FJ, et al. Toxicol Appl Pharmacol. 2001 Jun 15; 173(3):176–87.
Mercury concentrations in the human brain and kidneys in relation to exposure from dental amalgam fillings. Nylander M, et al. Swed Dent J. 1987; 11(5):179–87.

Multiple Sclerosis (MS)

A comparison of mental health of multiple sclerosis patients with silver/mercury dental fillings and those with fillings removed. Siblerud RL. Psychol Rep. 1992 Jun; 70(3 Pt 2):1139–51.

Cerebrospinal fluid protein changes in multiple sclerosis after dental amalgam removal. Huggins HA., et al. Altern Med Rev 1998;3:295–300.

Dental amalgam and multiple sclerosis: a case-control study in Montreal, Canada. Bangsi D., et al. Int J Epidemiol 1998;27:667–671.

Evidence that mercury from silver dental fillings may be an etiological factor in multiple sclerosis. Siblerud RL, et al. Sci Total Environ. 1994 Mar 15; 142 (3):191–205.

Mercury in cerebrospinal fluid in multiple sclerosis. Ahlrot-Westerlund B. Swed J Biol Med 1989;1:6–7.

Multiple sclerosis and dental amalgam: case-control study in Ferrara, Italy. Casetta I., et al. Neuroepidemiology 2001;20:134–137.

Multiple sclerosis, dental caries and fillings: a case-control study. McGrother CW., et al. Br Dent J 1999;187:261–264.

Theoretical considerations on the etiology of multiple sclerosis. Is multiple sclerosis a mercury allergy? Baasch E. Schweiz Arch Neurol Neurochir Psychiatr 1966;98:1–19.

Parkinson's Disease

Direct evidence for glutathione as mediator of apoptosis in neuronal cells. Nicole A, et al. Biomed Pharmacother. 1998; 52(9):349–55.

Epidemiologic Study on the Association between Body Burden Mercury Level and Idiopathic Parkinson's Disease. Ngim, C. Neuroepidemiology, 8:128–141 (1989).

Respiratory

Mercury—is it a respiratory tract allergen? Drouet M, et al. Allerg Immunol (Paris). 1990 Mar; 22(3):81, 84–8.

Thyroid

Effects of low mercury vapour exposure on the thyroid function in chloralkali workers. Ellingsen DG, et al. J Appl Toxicol. 2000 Nov-Dec; 20(6):483–9.

Vision

Color discrimination impairment in workers exposed to mercury vapor. Urban P, et al. Neurotoxicology. 2003 Aug; 24(4–5):711–6.

Reversible color vision loss in occupational exposure to metallic mercury. Cavalleri A, et al. Environ Res. 1998 May; 77(2):173–7.

Environmental release

Amalgam use and mercury emission in the Netherlands. Burger WG, et al. Ned Tijdschr Tandheelkd. 1997 Mar; 104(3):95–8.

Determination of methyl mercury in dental-unit wastewater. Stone ME., et al. Dent Mater 2003;19:675–679.

Mercury in the environment: a volatile problem. Lutter, Randall. Environment. Nov, 2002.

Mercury in the hair of crematoria workers. Maloney SR., et al. Lancet 1998;352:1602.

Mercury in saliva and the risk of exceeding limits for sewage in relation to exposure to amalgam fillings. Leistevuo J., et al. Arch Environ

More mercury from crematoria. Künzler P., et al. Nature 1991;349:746–747.

United States EPA International Mercury Market Study and the Role and Impact of US Environmental Policy 2004, referenced in Nov. 30, 2004 presentation by Linda Barr, EPA Office of Solid Waste, "EPA's Draft Mercury Use Reduction Program." www. epa.gov/region5/air/mercury/meetings/Nov04/barr.pdf.

Factors affecting release of mercury from amalgam fillings

Acid Conditions in Mouth

Dissolution of mercury from dental amalgam at different pH values. Marek M. J Dent Res. 1997 Jun; 76(6):1308–15.

Chewing and grinding

Influence of chewing gum consumption and dental contact of amalgam fillings to different metal restorations on urine mercury content. Gebel T, et al. Zentralbl Hyg Umweltmed. 1996 Nov; 199(1):69–75.

Intra-oral air mercury released from dental amalgam. Vimy MJ, et al. J Dent Res. 1985 Aug; 64(8):1069–71.

People with high mercury uptake from their own dental amalgam filling. Barregard L, et al. Occup Environ Med. 1995 Feb; 52(2):124–8.

Hot drinks

Factors influencing mercury evaporation rate from dental amalgam fillings. Bjorkman L, et al. Scand J Dent Res. 1992 Dec; 100(6):354–60.

Tooth brushing

Mercury exposure from dental fillings. II. Release and absorption. Langworth S, et al. Swed Dent J. 1988; 12(1–2):71–2.

Tooth grinding

The effect of dental amalgam restorations on blood mercury levels. Abraham JE, et al. J Dent Res. 1984 Jan; 63(1):71–3. 6582086 PubMed.

Impact of nocturnal bruxism on mercury uptake from dental amalgams. Isacsson G, et al. Eur J Oral Sci. 1997 Jun; 105 (3):251–7.

Fecal metals

Fecal Mercury. ISTERH Third International Conference and NTES Fourth Nordic Conference on Disease. Malmström C, et al. Stockholm (Huddinge), May 25–29, 1992.

Mercury in saliva and feces after removal of amalgam fillings. Bjorkman L, et al. Toxicol Appl Pharmacol. 1997 May; 144(1):156–62.

Fetus, baby, and child

Cognitive deficit in 7-year-old children with prenatal exposure to methylmercury. Grandjean P, et al. Neurotoxicol Teratol. 1997 Nov-Dec; 19(6):417–28.

Concentrations of heavy metals in maternal and umbilical cord blood. et al. Biometals. 1993 Spring; 6(1):61–6.

Continuing Increases in Autism Reported to California's Developmental Services System, Mercury in Retrograde Arch Gen Psychiatry. 2008;65(1):19–24.

Disposition of inhaled mercury vapor in pregnant rats: maternal toxicity and effects on developmental outcome. Morgan DL, et al. Toxicol Sci. 2002 Apr;66(2):261–73.

Environmental factors associated with a spectrum of neurodevelopmental deficits. Mendola P, et al. Ment Retard Dev Disabil Res Rev. 2002; 8(3):188–97.

Evolution of our understanding of methylmercury as a health threat. Watanabe C, et al. Environ Health Perspect. 1996 Apr; 104 Suppl 2:367–79.

Maternal amalgam dental fillings as the source of mercury exposure in developing fetus and newborn., Palkovicova L, et al. J Expo Sci Environ Epidemiol. 2007 Sep 12; Department of Environmental Medicine, Slovak Medical University, Bratislava, Slovakia.

Maternal-fetal distribution of mercury (203Hg) released from dental amalgam fillings. Vimy MJ, et al. Am J Physiol. 1990 Apr; 258(4 Pt 2):R939–45. www.ncbi.nlm.nih.gov/entrez/query.fcgi?cmd=Retrieve&db=pubmed&dopt=Abstract&list_uids=2331037.

Maternal-fetal transfer of metallic mercury via the placenta and milk. et al. Ann Clin Lab Sci. 1997 Mar-Apr; 27(2):135–41.

Mercury burden of human fetal and infant tissues. Drasch G, et al. Eur J Pediatr. 1994 Aug; 153(8):607–10.

Mercury in human colostrum and early breast milk. Its dependence on dental amalgam and other factors. Drasch G, et al. J Trace Elem Med Biol. 1998 Mar; 12(1):23–7.

Methyl mercury and inorganic mercury in Swedish pregnant women and in cord blood: influence of fish consumption. Bjornberg KA, et al. Environ Health Perspect. 2003 Apr; 111(4):637–41.

Placental transfer of mercury in pregnant rats which received dental amalgam restorations. Takahashi Y, et al. Toxicology. 2003 Mar 14; 185(1–2):23–33.

Technical report: mercury in the environment: implications for pediatricians. Goldman LR, et al. American Academy of Pediatrics: Committee on Environmental Health. Pediatrics. 2001 Jul; 108(1):197–205.

The effect of mercury vapour on cholinergic neurons in the fetal brain: studies on the expression of nerve growth factor and its low- and high-affinity receptors. Soderstrom S., et al. Brain Res Dev Brain Res 1995;85:96–108.

Fish and food

Evaluation of the dose of mercury in exposed and control subjects. Apostoli P, et al. Med Lav. 2002 May-Jun; 93(3):159–75.

Mercury in fish: cause for concern? U.S. Food and Drug Administration. FDA Consumer. September 1994. Revised May 1995.

Neurotoxicity of organomercurial compounds. Sanfeliu C, et al. Neurotox Res. 2003; 5(4):283–305.

Free radicals

Accumulation of mercury and its effect on antioxidant enzymes in brain, liver, and kidneys of mice. Hussain S, et al. J Environ Sci Health B. 1999 Jul;34(4):645–60.

Activated human T lymphocytes exhibit reduced susceptibility to methylmercury chloride-induced apoptosis. Close AH, et al. Toxicol Sci. 1999 May;49(1):68–77.

Mutagenicity of mercury chloride and mechanisms of cellular defence: the role of metal-binding proteins. Schurz F, et al. Mutagenesis. 2000 Nov; 15(6):525–30.

Oxidative mechanisms in the toxicity of metal ions. Stohs SJ, et al. Free Radic Biol Med. 1995 Feb; 18(2):321–36.

Toxic metals and oxidative stress part I: mechanisms involved in metal-induced oxidative damage. Ercal N, et al. Curr Top Med Chem. 2001 Dec; 1(6):529–39.

Galvanic and corrosion effects

Acceleration of corrosion of dental amalgam by abrasion. Marek M. J Dent Res. 1984 Jul; 63(7):1010–3.

Initial corrosion of amalgams in vitro. Brune D, et al. Scand J Dent Res. 1984 Apr; 92(2):165–71.

Unusual in vivo extensive corrosion of a low-silver amalgam restoration involving galvanic coupling: a case report. Toumelin-Chemla F, et al. Quintessence Int. 2003 Apr; 34(4):287–94.

Genetic/Mutations

Genotoxicity of mercury compounds. De Flora S, et al. Mutat Res. 1994 Feb; 317(1):57–79.

Lead and mercury mutagenesis: type of mutation dependent upon metal concentration. Ariza ME, et al. J Biochem Mol Toxicol. 1999; 13(2):107–12.

Mutagenesis of AS52 cells by low concentrations of lead (II) and mercury (II). Ariza ME, et al. Environ Mol Mutagen. 1996; 27(1):30–3.

Hair analysis

The present mercury contents of scalp hair and clinical symptoms in inhabitants of the Minamata area. Harada M, et al. Environ Res. 1998 May; 77(2):160–4.

Health, general

Environmental medicine, part three: long-term effects of chronic low-dose mercury exposure. Crinnion WJ. Altern Med Rev. 2000 Jun; 5(3):209–23.

Removal of dental amalgam and other metal alloys supported by antioxidant therapy alleviates symptoms and improves quality of life in patients with amalgam-associated ill health. Lindh U, et al. Neuroendocrinol Lett. 2002 Oct–Dec; 23(5–6):459–82.

Immune system, autoimmune and allergy

Activation of the immune system and systemic immune-complex deposits in Brown Norway rats with dental amalgam restorations. Hultman P, et al. J Dent Res 1998;77:1415–1425.

Adverse immunological effects and autoimmunity induced by dental amalgam and alloy in mice. Hultman P, et al. FASEB J. 1994 Nov; 8(14):1183–90.

Amalgames dentaires et allergie. Veron C, Hildebrand HF, Martin P. J Biol Buccale 1986;14:83–100.

Contact dermatitis due to the mercury of amalgam dental fillings. Robinson, H.M., Bereston, E.S. Arch Dermatol Syphilol. 59:116–8, 1949.

Dental amalgam as one of the risk factors in autoimmune diseases. Bartova J, et al. Neuroendocrinol Lett. 2003 Feb-Apr; 24(1–2):65–7.

Development of mercury hypersensitivity among dental students. White, R.R., Brandt, R.L. J Amer Dent Assoc. 92:1204–7, 1976.

Direct and indirect restorative materials. J Am Dent Assoc, vol 134, no 4, 463–472. © 2003.

Does amalgam affect the immune system? A controversial issue. Enestrom S, et al. Int Arch Allergy Immunol. 1995 Mar; 106(3):180–203.

Effects of mercury on human polymorphonuclear leukocyte function in vitro. Contrino J, et al. Am J Pathol. 1988 Jul; 132(1):110–8.

Epidemiologic Study of Occupational Contact Dermatitis in the Dental Clinic. D.Kawahara et al. Contact Dermatitis, vol 28, no.2, pp114–5,1993.

Immunoglobulin levels in workers exposed to inorganic mercury. Queiroz ML, et al. Pharmacol Toxicol. 1994 Feb; 74(2):72–5.

Immunological and Brain MRI Changes in Patients with Suspected Metal Intoxication. Tibbling L, et al. International Journal of Occupational Medicine and Toxicology. vol. 4. no. 2. 1995.

Immunotoxic effects of mercuric compounds on human lymphocytes and monocytes. II. Alterations in cell viability. Shenker BJ, et al. Immunopharmacol Immunotoxicol. 1992; 14(3):555–77.

Mercury-specific lymphocytes: an indication of mercury allergy in man. Stejskal VD., et al. J Clin Immunol 1996;16:31–40.

Mercury and nickel allergy: risk factors in fatigue and autoimmunity. Stejskal VD, et al. Neuroendocrinol Lett 1999;20:221–228.

Metal-specific lymphocytes: biomarkers of sensitivity in man. Stejskal VD, et al. Neuroendocrinol Lett 1999;20:289–298.

Murine mercury-induced autoimmunity: a model of chemically related autoimmunity in humans. Bagenstose LM, et al. Immunol Res. 1999; 20(1):67–78.

Oral Contact Allergies. Source: Special Report By: Wayne Kuznar. Originally published: June 1, 2003; http://socalphys.mediwire.com/main/Default.aspx?P=Content&ArticleID=60932.

Oral exposure to inorganic mercury alters T lymphocyte phenotypes and cytokine expression in BALB/c mice. Kim SH, et al. Arch Toxicol. 2003 Aug 20.

Oral Lichenoid lesions caused by allergy to mercury in amalgam fillings. Bryan K. Pang, et al. Contact & Occupational Dermatitis Clinic, Skin & Cancer Foundation, NSW, 2010, Australia. Contact Dermatitis 33 (6), 423–427. doi:10.1111/j.1600–0536.1995. tb02079.x.

Oral lichen planus and allergy to dental amalgam restorations. Laeijendecker R, Dekker SK, Burger PM, Mulder PG, Van Joost T, Neumann MH. Arch Dermatol. 2004 Dec;140(12):1434–8.

Oral lichen planus and contact allergy to mercury. Finne, K., et al. Int J Oral Surg 11 (1982), 236–239.

Prevalence of mercury hypersensitivity among dental students. E.G. Miller et al. J Dent Res. 64:Abstract 1472, p338, 1985.

Prevalences of positive skin test responses to 10 common allergens in the US population: Results from the Third National Health and Nutrition Examination Survey. Arbes SJ et al. J Allergy Clin Immunol. 2005; 116:377–383.

Systemic Autoimmunity Due to Mercury Vapor Exposure in Genetically Susceptible Mice: Dose-Response Studies. Warfvinge, et al. Toxicol Appl Pharmacol, 132:299–309 (1995).

The beneficial effects of amalgam replacement on health of patients with autoimmunity. Stejskal VDM, et al. Neuroendocrinol Lett 2004; 25: 211–218.

The health and economic impact of rhinitis. A roundtable discussion. Stempel DA. Am J Manag Care. 1997;3:S8-S18.

The role of metals in autoimmunity and the link to neuroendocrinology. Stejskal VD, et al Neuroendocrinol Lett 1999;20:351–364.

The possibilities of allergic reactions from silver amalgam restorations. Djerassi, E., Berova, N. Int Dent J. 19:48l-8, 1969.

Validity of MELISA® for metal sensitivity testing. Valentine-Thon E., et al. Neuroendocrinol Lett 2003;24:57–64.

Infertility and birth defects

Effect of heavy metals on immune reactions in patients with infertility. Stejskal VD., et al. Cas Lek Cesk. 2003;142:285–288.

Effect of occupational exposures on male fertility: literature review. Sheiner EK.., et al. Ind Health 2003;41:55–62.

Heavy metals and fertility. Gerhard I, et al. J Toxicol Environ Health A. 1998 Aug 21; 54(8):593–611.

Impact of heavy metals on hormonal and immunological factors in women with repeated miscarriages. Gerhard I, et al. Hum Reprod Update. 1998 May-Jun; 4(3):301–9.

Infertility and Birth Defects: Is Mercury from Dental Fillings a Hidden Cause? Ziff S, et al. Bio-Probe, Inc. ISBN: 0–941011–03–8. 1987.

Paternal exposure to mercury and spontaneous abortions. Cordier S, et al. Br J Ind Med. 1991 Jun; 48(6):375–81.

The effect of occupational exposure to mercury vapour on the fertility of female dental assistants. Rowland AS., et al. Occup Environ Med 1994;51:28–34.

Intestinal

Association of mercury resistance with antibiotic resistance in the gram-negative fecal bacteria of primates. Wireman, J. et al. Applied Environmental Microbiology, 63/11: 4494–4503, Nov 1997. aem.asm.org/cgi/content/abstract/63/11/4494.

Bacterial mercury resistance from atoms to ecosystems. Barkay T, et al. FEMS Microbiol Rev. 2003 Jun; 27(2–3):355–84.

Mercury released from dental "silver" fillings provokes an increase in mercury and antibiotic resistant bacteria in primates oral and intestinal flora. Vimy, M.J., et al. Antimicrobial Agents and Chemotherapy, 37: 825–834, 1993. www.ncbi.nlm.nih.gov/entrez/query.fcgi?cmd=Retrieve&db=pubmed&dopt=Abstract&list_uids=8280208.

Legal and political

The science and politics of dental amalgam. Gelband H. Int J Technol Assess Health Care. 1998 Winter; 14(1):123–34.

UN Committee Recommends Stricter Mercury Limits. New York, June 30, 2003. Environment News Service (ENS).

Dentists Settle in Mercury Cleanup Case. American Dental Association News. Aug. 15, 1988.

Methylation

Biosynthesis of methylmercury compounds by the intestinal flora of the rat. Rowland I, et al. Arch Environ Health. 1977 Jan-Feb; 32(1):24–8.

Methylation of mercury from dental amalgam and mercuric chloride by oral streptococci in vitro. Heintze U, et al. Scand J Dent Res. 1983 Apr; 91(2):150–2.

The methylation of mercuric chloride by human intestinal bacteria. Rowland IR, et al. Experientia. 1975 SEP 15; 31(9):1064–5.

Transformations of inorganic mercury by Candida albicans and Saccharomyces cerevisiae. Yannai S, et al. Appl Environ Microbiol. 1991 Jan; 57(1):245–7.

Oral

An amalgam tattoo causing local and systemic disease? Weaver T, et al. Oral Surg Oral Med Oral Pathol. 1987 Jan; 63(1):137–40.

Mercury in saliva and feces after removal of amalgam fillings. Bjorkman L, et al. Toxicol Appl Pharmacol. 1997 May; 144(1):156–62.

The relationship between mercury from dental amalgam and oral cavity health. Siblerud RL. Ann Dent. 1990 Winter; 49(2):6–10.

Periodontal

Maternal periodontitis and prematurity. Part I: Obstetric outcome of prematurity and growth restriction. Offenbacher S, et al. Ann Periodontol. 2001 Dec; 6(1):164–74.

Periodontal disease and cardiovascular disease: epidemiology and possible mechanisms. Genco R, et al. J Am Dent Assoc. 2002 Jun; 133 Suppl:14S-22S.

Periodontal disease is associated with lower antioxidant capacity in whole saliva and evidence of increased protein oxidation. Sculley DV, et al. Clin Sci (Lond). 2003 Aug; 105(2):167–72.

Relationship between periodontal disease and C-reactive protein among adults in the Atherosclerosis Risk in Communities study. Slade GD, et al. Arch Intern Med. 2003 May 26; 163(10):1172–9.

Release and absorption

Absorption

Compositions of surface layers formed on amalgams in air, water, and saline. Hanawa T, et al. Dent Mater J. 1993 Dec; 12(2):118–26.

Daily dose estimates of mercury from dental amalgams. Lorscheider FL, et al. J Dent Res. 1991 Mar; 70(3):233–7.

Distribution of mercury in various tissues of guinea-pigs after application of dental amalgam fillings (a pilot study). Fredin B. Sci Total Environ. 1987 Oct; 66:263–8.

Documented clinical side-effects to dental amalgam. Ziff MF. Adv Dent Res. 1992 Sep; 6:131–4.

Estimation of mercury body burden from dental amalgam: computer stimulation of a metabolic compartmental model. Vimy MJ, et al. J Dent Res. 1986 Dec; 65(12):1415–9.

Estimation of the uptake of mercury from amalgam fillings based on urinary excretion of mercury in Swedish subjects. Weiner JA, et al. Sci Total Environ. 1995 Jun 30; 168(3):255–65.

Long-term mercury excretion in urine after removal of amalgam fillings. Begerow J, et al. Int Arch Occup Environ Health. 1994; 66(3):209–12.

Mercury in Biological Fluids After Amalgam Removal, Sandborgh-Englund, et al., J Dent Res, 77(4): 615–24 (Apr. 1998).

Mercury Exposure from Silver Tooth Fillings: Emerging Evidence Questions a Traditional Dental Paradigm, Lorscheider, FL; et al., FASEB J., 9:504–8 (1995).

Side-effects: mercury contribution to body burden from dental amalgam. Reinhardt JW. Adv Dent Res. 1992 Sep; 6:110–3.

Silver amalgam: An unstable material. Malmström C, et al. Danish Dental Journal. Tidsskr. f. Tandlaeger. October 1989. Swedish paper translated by Mats Hansson Ph.D., in Bio-Probe Newsletter. Vol 9(1):5–6. Jan. 1993.

Urinary mercury after administration of 2, 3-dimercaptopropane-1-sulfonic acid: correlation with dental amalgam score. Aposhian HV, et al. FASEB J. 1992 Apr; 6(7):2472–6.

Release

A case of high mercury exposure from dental amalgam. Langworth S, et al. Eur J Oral Sci. 1996 Jun; 104(3):320–1.

A study of the release of mercury vapor from different types of amalgam alloys. A.Berglund, J Dent Res, 1993, 72:939–946.

Exposure to mercury in the population. II. Mercury release from amalgam fillings. Zander D, et al. Zentralbl Hyg Umweltmed. 1990 Oct; 190(4):325–34.

Human exposure to mercury and silver released from dental amalgam restorations. Skare I, et al. Arch Environ Health. 1994 Sep-Oct; 49(5):384–94.

Influence of amalgam fillings on Hg levels and total antioxidant activity in plasma of healthy donors. Pizzichini M, et al. Sci Total Environ. 2003 Jan 1; 301(1–3):43–50.

Influence of liquid films on mercury vapor loss from dental amalgam. Mahler DB, et al. Dent Mater. 2002 Jul; 18(5):407–12.

Inhalation of Mercury-Contaminated Particulate Matter by Dentists: An Overlooked Occupational Risk, Richardson, G.M.,Human and Ecological Risk Assessment, 9:1519–1531 (2003).

Intra-oral air mercury released from dental amalgam. Vimy MJ, et al. J Dent Res. 1985 Aug; 64(8):1069–71.

Mercury concentration in the mouth mucosa of patients with amalgam fillings. Willershausen-Zonnchen B, et al. Dtsch Med Wochenschr. 1992 Nov 13; 117(46):1743–7.

Mercury in saliva and feces after removal of amalgam fillings. Bjorkman L, et al. Toxicol Appl Pharmacol. 1997 May; 144(1):156–62.

Mercury vapor in the oral cavity in relation to the number of amalgam fillings and chronic mercury poisoning. H. Lichtenberg. Journal of Orthomolecular Medicine, 1996, 11:2, 87–94.

Mercury vaporization from amalgams with varied alloy composition. Ferracane J L, et al., J Dent Res 1995; 74:1414–1417.

Model of mercury vapor transport from amalgam restorations in the oral cavity. Olsson S, et al. J Dent Res. 1989 Mar; 68(3):504–8.

Serial measurements of intra-oral air mercury: estimation of daily dose from dental amalgam. Vimy MJ, et al. J Dent Res. 1985 Aug; 64(8):1072–5.

Relationship to amalgam fillings

Factors affecting internal mercury burdens among eastern German children. Trepka MJ, et al. Arch Environ Health. 1997 Mar-Apr; 52(2):134–8.

Mercury in biological fluids after amalgam removal. Sandborgh-Englund G, et al J. J Dent Res. 1998 Apr; 77(4):615–24.

Mercury concentrations in the human brain and kidneys in relation to exposure from dental amalgam fillings. Nylander M, et al. Swed Dent J. 1987; 11(5):179–87.

Resistance to antibiotics

Mercury released from dental "silver" fillings provokes an increase in mercury- and antibiotic-resistant bacteria in oral and intestinal floras of primates. Summers AO, et al. Antimicrob Agents Chemother. 1993 Apr; 37(4):825–34.

Resistance of the normal human microflora to mercury and antimicrobials after exposure to mercury from dental amalgam fillings. Edlund C, et al. Clin Infect Dis. 1996 Jun; 22(6):944–50.

Role of mercury (Hg) in resistant infections & effective treatment of Chlamydia trachomatis and Herpes family viral infections (and potential treatment for cancer) by removing localized Hg deposits with Chinese parsley and delivering effective antibiotics using various drug uptake enhancement methods. Omura Y, et al. Acupunct Electrother Res. 1995 Aug-Dec; 20(3–4):195–229.

Safety

World Health Organization, Environmental Health Criteria 118: Inorganic Mercury (1991) p. 36.

Stimulation

Exposure to mercury vapor during setting, removing, and polishing amalgam restorations. Haikel Y, et al. J Biomed Mater Res. 1990 Nov; 24(11):1551–8.

Symptoms

ABC on mercury poisoning from dental amalgam fillings. Handbook for victims of mercury-poisoning from dental amalgam. Swedish Association of Dental Mercury Patients. Nov 1993. Mats Hanson, Ph.D.

Adverse health effects related to mercury exposure from dental amalgam fillings: toxicological or psychological causes? Bailer J, et al. Psychol Med. 2001 Feb; 31(2):255–63.

Changes in the nervous system due to occupational metallic mercury poisoning. Langauer-Lewowicka H, et al. Neurol Neurochir Pol. 1997 Sep-Oct; 31(5):905–13.

Mercury: major issues in environmental health. Clarkson TW. Environ Health Perspect. 1993 Apr; 100:31–8.

Mercury vapour in the oral cavity in relation to the number of amalgam surfaces and the classic symptoms. Lichtenberg H. Journal of Orthomolecular Medicine Vol 11:2. 87–94 1996.

Physical and mental problems attributed to dental amalgam fillings: a descriptive study of 99 self-referred patients compared with 272 controls. Malt UF, et al. Psychosom Med. 1997 Jan-Feb; 59(1):32–41.

Relationship between mercury from dental amalgam and health. Siblerud RL. Toxic Substances Journal. 10:425–444 1990b.

Symptoms improvement after amalgam removal

A multicenter survey of amalgam fillings and subjective complaints in non-selected patients in the dental practice. Melchart D., et al. Eur J Oral Sci 1998;106:770–777.

Adverse health effects related to mercury exposure from dental amalgam fillings: toxicological or psychological causes? Bailer J., et al. Psychol Med 2001;31:255–263.

Amalgam. XII. Amalgam removed and patient cured. Eijkman MA, et al. Ned Tijdschr Tandheelkd. 1994 Feb; 101(2):50–3.

Commentary regarding the article by Gottwald et al.: "Amalgam disease"—poisoning, allergy, or psychic disorder? Mutter J., et al. Int J Hyg Environ Health 2003;206:69–70.

Consolidated symptoms of 1, 569 patients. Ziff S. Bio-Probe Newsletter. 9:2. March 1993.

Dental Amalgam and Health Experience: Exploring Health Outcomes and Issues for People Medically Diagnosed with Mercury Poisoning. Jones L. The Bulletin of the New Zealand Psychological Society. 97, 29–33. 1999.

Elimination of symptoms by removal of dental amalgam from mercury poisoned patients, as compared with a control group of average patients. Lichtenberg HJ. Journal of Orthomolecular Medicine. 1993; 8: pp.145–148.

Psychological and somatic subjective symptoms as a result of dermatological patch testing with metallic mercury and phenyl mercuric acetate. Marcusson JA. Toxicol Lett 1996;84:113–122.

Relationship between mercury from dental amalgam and mental health. Am J Psychother. Siblerud RL.1989 Oct; 43(4):575–87.

Removal of dental amalgam and other metal alloys supported by antioxidant therapy alleviates symptoms and improves quality of life in patients with amalgam-associated ill health. Lindh U, et al. Neuroendocrinol Lett. 2002 Oct–Dec; 23(5–6):459–82.

Results of dental amalgam removal and mercury detoxification using DMPS and neural therapy. Kidd RF. Altern Ther Health Med. 2000 Jul; 6(4):49–55.

Symptoms before and after proper amalgam removal in relation to serum-globulin reaction to metals. Lichtenberg HJ. Orthomolec Med 1996:11:195–204. www.lichtenberg.dk/symptoms_before_and_after_proper.htm.

Toxicity

Correlation of dental amalgam with mercury in brain tissue. Eggleston DW, et al. J Prosthet Dent. 1987 Dec; 58(6):704–7.

Dental amalgam: a review of the literature. Eggleston DW. Compendium. 1989 Sep; 10(9):500–5.

Dental mercury—a public health hazard. Pleva J. Rev Environ Health. 1994 Jan-Mar; 10(1):1–27.

Does mercury from amalgam restorations constitute a health hazard? Weiner JA, et al. Sci Total Environ. 1990 Dec 1; 99(1–2):1–22.

Environmental exposure to mercury and its toxicopathologic implications for public health. Tchounwou PB, et al. Environ Toxicol. 2003 Jun; 18(3):149–75.

Environmental medicine, part three: long-term effects of chronic low-dose mercury exposure. Crinnion WJ. Altern Med Rev. 2000 Jun;5(3):209–23.

Evaluation of the safety issue of mercury release from dental fillings. Lorscheider FL, et al. FASEB J. 1993 Dec; 7(15):1432–3.

Mercury exposure and early effects: an overview. Kazantzis G. Med Lav. 2002 May–Jun; 93(3):139–47.

Mercury exposure from "silver" tooth fillings: emerging evidence questions a traditional dental paradigm. Lorscheider FL, et al. FASEB J. 1995 Apr; 9(7):504–8.

Mercury exposure from "silver" fillings. Lorscheider FL, et al. Lancet. 1991 May 4; 337(8749):1103.

Metals and Neurotoxic Effects: Cytotoxicity of Selected Metallic Compounds on Chick Ganglia Cultures, Sharma, RP, et al. J Comp Pathol, 91(2):235–44 (1981).

Organic mercury compounds: human exposure and its relevance to public health. Risher JF, et al. Toxicol Ind Health. 2002 Apr; 18(3):109–60.

Side-effects: mercury contribution to body burden from dental amalgam. Reinhardt JW. Adv Dent Res. 1992 Sep; 6:110–3.

The dental amalgam issue. A review. Hanson M, et al. Experientia. 1991 Jan 15; 47(1):9–22.

The relationship between mercury concentration in human organs and different predictor variables. Weiner JA, et al. Sci Total Environ. 1993 Sep 30; 138(1–3):101–15.

Toxicity of mercury. Langford N, et al. J Hum Hypertens. 1999 Oct;13(10):651–6.

Toxicology of mercury. Clarkson TW. Crit Rev Clin Lab Sci. 1997 Aug; 34(4):369–403.

Whole-body imaging of the distribution of mercury released from dental fillings into monkey tissues. Hahn LJ, et al. FASEB J. 1990 Nov; 4(14):3256–60.

Transportation

Transport of toxic metals by molecular mimicry. Ballatori N. Environ Health Perspect. 2002 Oct; 110 Suppl 5:689–94.

Types of amalgam fillings

Effect of selenium on mercury vapour released from dental amalgams: an in vitro study. Psarras V, et al. Swed Dent J. 1994;18(1–2):15–23.

WHO: No safe level of Hg

World Health Organization (WHO), Environmental Health Criteria 118: Inorganic Mercury, pp, 28–33, 84–113, Geneva, 1991.

Inorganic Mercury. WHO Environmental Health Criteria 118.

WHO Geneva. 1991. ISBN 92-4-157118-7.

Glossary

activated charcoal   A carbon material that is able to bind to poisons and toxins, including mercury, in the intestine and prevent their absorption into the body.

acute poisoning   A large one-time dose of a poisonous substance that can be fatal.

Agency for Toxic Substances and Disease Registry (ATSDR)   ATSDR is directed by congressional mandate to perform specific functions concerning the effect on public health of hazardous substances in the environment.

Acquired Immune Deficiency Syndrome (AIDS)   A collection of symptoms and infections resulting from damage to the immune system caused by the human immunodeficiency virus (HIV).

allergen   A substance that is capable of causing an immune system reaction. Common allergens are dusts, pollens, dander, food, and mercury.

allergy   The actual physical reaction the body experiences to an allergen. Common reactions include rash, itching, sneezing, coughing, and abdominal pain.

alpha lipoic acid (ALA)   Also known as thioctic acid, ALA has many roles. It helps the body produce energy, is a potent antioxidant, and can chelate (remove) mercury from the body.

amalgam filling   An alloy resulting from the mixing of mercury with one or more metals, most commonly silver, copper, tin, and zinc.

amalgamation   The mixing of different metals. A mercury amalgam filling is an amalgamation of mercury, silver, copper, tin, and zinc.

ambient mercury   An extremely small amount of mercury that's naturally present in the environment.

American Dental Association (ADA)   A professional member-based association of dentists founded in 1859.

American Society of Dental Surgeons (ASDS)   Physician-dentists established the ASDS in 1840. The first national dental association in America, the purpose of ASDS was to ban the use of mercury amalgam fillings.

amino acids   Amino acids are molecules that contain both amine and carboxyl groups. When they are joined together they make proteins, enzymes, and antioxidants. There are 20 amino acids that that are essential to sustain life.

anecdotal evidence   Evidence based on the subjective experiences of individuals rather than on objective scientific evidence.

antioxidant   A substance that protects the body against mercury, free radicals, and other harmful substances. Antioxidants are the key ingredient of the immune and detoxification systems. Important antioxidants are glutathione (GSH), alpha lipoic acid (ALA), beta-carotene (a vitamin A precursor), vitamin C, vitamin E, and selenium.

apoptosis   A process by which a cell programs its own death. It is believed that this takes place because the cell is under so much stress that it can no longer survive and, in effect, commits suicide.

atom   The smallest part of an element that still retains its unique characteristics.

autism   A complex learning and developmental disorder that typically appears during the first three years of life. Its symptoms mimic those of early chronic mercury poisoning.

autoimmune   A reaction that occurs when the immune system does not recognize its own cells and tissues and initiates an immune response. If this response is long-lasting, an autoimmune disease can result.

barber-dentist   A barber, metal worker, wood worker, or other tradesman who also filled and extracted teeth in the 1800s.

Bernard, Sallie   Co-founder and executive director of SafeMinds, a private non-profit organization founded to investigate and raise awareness of the risks to infants and children of exposure to mercury from medical products, including thimerosal in vaccines.

biocompatible dental materials   Dental materials that don't induce harmful reactions in or on the body.

biocompatibility testing   Biocompatibility testing is done to determine the body's response to a material it will be in contact with, such as a dental filling .

Bisphenol A   A monomer and a key ingredient in the manufacturing of plastic and resins, including dental composites.

blood brain barrier   A system of microscopic blood vessels only a single cell thick that allows some substances to pass into the brain and prevent others from entering.

blood mercury test   A test that accurately detects mercury levels found in the blood at the time the blood is drawn.

Candida   A yeast infection that can cause numerous digestive, general, and neurological problems. Chronic exposure to mercury can make it resistant to treatment.

cavitation   An area in the jawbone that has not properly healed after a tooth extraction, which can contain toxins and bacteria. A cavitation is also referred to as neuralgia-inducing cavitational osteonecrosis (NICO).

Centers for Disease Control and Prevention (CDC)   An agency of the federal Department of Health and Human Services located in Atlanta, Georgia. Its stated mission is "to promote health and quality of life by preventing and controlling disease, injury, and disability."

central nervous system (CNS)   The portion of the human nervous system that consists of the brain, spinal cord and their nerve endings. Collectively, they serve as the center that regulates the body's reaction to stimulus.

CEREC   An innovative system used to manufacture ceramic restorations, inlays, onlays, and crowns, in one office visit.

chelator   A material that binds with various substances, both harmful and necessary, and facilitates their removal from the body. Chelators can be natural, such as chlorella, or manufactured by drug companies. Antioxidants produced by the body, such as glutathione, also act as chelators.

composite filling   A combination of glass fillers and plastic resin material. This mixture is light-sensitive and hardens or "cures" when a special light is applied to the mixture. Composite fillings are a safe alternative to amalgam fillings.

contact point   The point at which two adjacent teeth touch.

chronic mercury poisoning   Poisoning that results from continual exposure to small amounts of mercury over a long period of time.

chunking   Removing amalgam fillings in sections to minimize heating the filling and reduce mercury vapor release.

Crawcours brothers   Two French brothers who introduced amalgam fillings to England in 1830 and to America in 1833.

cysteine   One of only two amino acids that have a sulfhydryl group. Cysteine is a component of glutathione, which is able to chelate and remove mercury from the body.

Dental Amalgam Mercury Solutions (DAMS)   A patient support group providing information to mercury toxic individuals on testing and treatment options, and also features a list of specially trained dentists and doctors.

dental board   A state agency that regulates the dental profession in that state and has the power to bestow and revoke licenses to practice dentistry. Its decisions generally reflect ADA standards and positions.

dental disease   Tooth decay, gum disease, and other oral infections. Gum disease is the more serious, and although it begins in the mouth, if left unchecked it can contribute to more serious diseases that can negatively affect quality of life and shorten life expectancy.

Dental Wellness Institute   Founded in 1997 by Dr. Tom McGuire with the goal of educating the public about the relationship of oral to overall health and bridging the gap between the dental and medical professions.

detoxification pathway   A term that refers to the various routes the body uses to eliminate what it wants to remove. Feces, urine, skin, hair, lungs, and nails are detoxification pathways.

detoxification system   The liver, kidneys, and other organs responsible for eliminating toxic substances, such as mercury, from the body.

direct composite   A composite filling is mixture of plastic and glass that is done in one appointment. Most often used for smaller cavities. See *composite filling.*

DMPS   2,3-dimercapto-1-propane sulfonic acid is a pharmaceutical chelator, which has not yet received final FDA approval. It can aggressively remove mercury from the body via the kidneys. Usually administered intravenously and requires a prescription.

DMSA   Dimercaptosuccinic acid is a pharmaceutical chelator that can aggressively remove mercury from the body via the kidneys. Usually taken orally and requires a prescription.

doctor-dentists   Physicians who also practiced dentistry in the early 1800s.

Electro-Dermal screening (EDS)   This computer-based instrument measures the energy of the body, including detecting allergies and sensitivities to many materials. It is a form of biofeedback.

elemental mercury   Mercury in its pure liquid form. This is the second most toxic form of mercury and is the type of mercury used in amalgam fillings. At room temperature, elemental mercury is odorless and invisible and releases mercury atoms as a poisonous vapor. The amount of mercury vapor released from elemental mercury increases in direct proportion to the temperature it is heated to.

environmental exposure   Exposure to a toxic substance from the environment (air, water, and soil).

Environmental Protection Agency (EPA)   The federal agency responsible for protecting human health and safeguarding the natural environment. In 1988, the EPA labeled the components of dental amalgam and scrap dental amalgam as a toxic waste material. Under this regulation, both must be placed in a hazardous waste container.

enzyme   Made of amino acids, enzymes are essential to health. Every chemical reaction in the body requires a specific enzyme, and every enzyme is necessary for optimal health.

fecal metals test   A test that detects mercury and other heavy metals in the feces.

Food and Drug Administration (FDA)   An agency of the U.S. Department of Health and Human Services. Responsible for regulating foods, dietary supplements, drugs, vaccines, biological medical products, blood products, medical devices, radiation-emitting devices, veterinary products, and cosmetics.

free radicals   Molecules that contain at least one unpaired electron and are known to damage healthy cells. To complete their own electronic structure, free radicals steal electrons from intact molecules, which generate new free radicals, which then react with other molecules. Free radicals are extremely toxic to the body and severely stress the immune system.

galvanic current   A battery-like current that flows between a high noble metal filling, such as gold, to a low noble metal, such as mercury in amalgam fillings. This current causes the release of mercury from amalgam fillings.

general body   For the purposes of this book, the general body includes every part of the body except the brain and central nervous system.

glutathione   The "king" of antioxidants, glutathione (GSH) is manufactured by the body, neutralizes free radicals, and has primary responsibility for removing mercury from the body. If levels of glutathione are sufficient, the immune system can eliminate significant amounts of mercury. If glutathione levels decrease, the body is less effective in this important function.

hair analysis   A test to determine the amounts of mineral and trace elements, including mercury, in the hair.

half-life   The time required for half the amount of a radioactive substance to decay.

heavy metal   Any metallic element that has a high density and is poisonous in small amounts. Heavy metals include mercury, arsenic, cadmium, chromium, and lead.

heavy metal synergism   The total effect of two or more metals on the body, which is greater than the sum of the effects of the individual metals. Mercury, arsenic, cadmium, and lead all exhibit synergism, especially when lead and mercury are present together.

hemoglobin   The iron-containing protein in red blood cells that transports oxygen to the body.

Human Immunodeficiency Virus (HIV)   This type of retrovirus can lead to acquired immune deficiency syndrome (AIDS), a condition in which the immune system fails, leading to numerous life-threatening infections.

Holistic Dental Association (HAD)   A holistic dental organization dedicated to teaching concerned dentists about the value of healthy dentistry.

Holmes, Amy   A physician and world-renowned practitioner of oral chelation for children who show evidence of mercury poisoning. She helped pioneer a new direction in mercury detoxification of children, based on careful attention to testing and nutrient/mineral supplementation.

immune system   The function of the immune system is to protect the body by neutralizing free radicals and eliminating bacteria, viruses, fungi, and poisonous and toxic substances, including mercury and other heavy metals.

indirect composites   A composite filling that requires two visits and is made at a dental laboratory.

inorganic mercury   The least toxic form of mercury. Inorganic mercury is chemically bonded in compounds with other elements (except carbon). Mercuric chloride is an example of an inorganic mercury compound.

Institute of Nutritional Dentistry (IND)   An organization that provides dentists with access to the latest information on all aspects of nutritional dentistry, including innovative technology, products, and biocompatible dental materials.

International Academy of Oral Medicine and Toxicology (IAOMT)   A science-based organization for dental, medical, and research professionals who seek to promote mercury free dentistry and raise the standards of health and material biocompatibility in the dental practice. One of the IAOMT's most recognized accomplishment is its development of a protocol for the safe removal of mercury amalgam fillings.

International Academy of Biological Dentistry and Medicine (IABDM)   An organization of dentists, scientists, and health practitioners that researches alternative treatments and materials that can be incorporated into the dental practice to help improve oral and overall health.

International Association of Mercury Free Dentists   An association of dedicated mercury free dentists who commit to practicing mercury safe dentistry.

lichen planus   Common chronic inflammatory disease of the oral mucous membranes that is sometimes painful. Lichen planus of the mucosa may lead to oral cancer, particularly when there's chronic exposure to a toxic substance, such as mercury.

kinesiology   A subjective method of testing the body for substances it may not be compatible with. Also referred to as "muscle testing."

Mad Hatter's disease   Neurological and other symptoms of mercury toxicity that hat makers (hatters) suffered in the 19th century as a result of using elemental mercury to produce felt for hats.

MELISA® test   A test that measures the reactivity of white blood cells to a number of metals, including mercury. It determines sensitivity to metals by placing a range of metals into contact with white blood cells and monitoring the reaction.

mercurochrome   A household first aid solution that millions of people once applied to cuts. Mercurochrome is now banned because of its mercury content.

mercury   The most poisonous naturally-occurring nonradioactive substance on earth. Mercury is many times more toxic than arsenic, lead, or cadmium. There are three types of mercury: elemental, inorganic, and organic. While all forms of mercury are extremely toxic, organic mercury is the most toxic, followed closely by elemental, and then inorganic.

mercury amalgam fillings   Also known as silver fillings or amalgam fillings mercury amalgam filling is a mixture of various metals and consists of 50 percent elemental mercury.

mercury contaminated fish   Fish, mostly large ocean fish, that have been shown to have high levels of poisonous organic mercury.

mercury detoxification   The process of removing mercury from the body.

mercury free dentists   Dentists who do not place mercury amalgam (silver) fillings.

mercury safe dentists   Dentists who believe mercury amalgam (silver) fillings are a health hazard, do not use amalgams, and use a safe removal protocol designed minimize a patient's exposure to mercury during amalgam removal.

mercury poisoning   Exposure to mercury that results in a variety of symptoms, including tremors, anxiety, heart disease, memory loss, autoimmune disease, and depression.

mercury vapor   Highly poisonous mercury that is released as a vapor from elemental mercury.

Jerome mercury vapor analyzer   The instrument most often used to test for mercury vapor in the workplace.

metal free dentists   Dentists who do not put any metal filling material in, or on, teeth.

methionine   An important amino acid that has a sulfhydryl group.

methyl mercury The most common form of organic mercury. It occurs when elemental mercury is converted to organic mercury by microorganisms.

microgram (mcg) The smallest unit of weight commonly used. It weighs 1000 times less than a milligram (mg). There are 1000 milligrams in a gram (g). (For reference, there are 28.35 grams in an ounce.)

micronize To reduce subtances to particles that are only a few microns in diameter.

muscle testing A method that alternative health practitioners use to test a person's response to stress, including materials that could cause an allergic reaction. Also referred to as "Kinesiology. "

mutagenic substance A physical or chemical agent that changes the genetic information (usually DNA) of an organism.

National Institute for Occupational Safety and Health (NIOSH) The federal agency responsible for conducting research and making recommendations for the prevention of work-related disease and injury.

Natural Cellular Defense (NCD) A zeolite product derived from natural volcanic minerals. Its honeycomb framework (similar to cages) works at the cellular level to trap heavy metals and toxins and safely remove them from the body.

Natural Detox Factors (NDF) A chlorella product that is micronized so it can be assimilated in the intestine. It has been shown to be able to remove mercury via the kidneys.

neurotoxin A toxic agent or substance that inhibits, damages, or destroys the tissues of the nervous system, especially neurons, the conducting cells of the body's central nervous system.

night guard A product that fits in the mouth and protects those who grind their teeth from tooth-to-filling or filling-to-filling contact. Night guards are soft or hard and can significantly reduce exposure to mercury vapor from amalgam fillings for those who grind their teeth.

noble metal filling A metal or alloy, such as gold, that is resistant to oxidation and corrosion.

occlusal contact Contact between opposing surfaces of the teeth, or contact between the grinding or biting surfaces of the teeth.

occupational exposure Exposure to a toxic substances at the workplace.

Occupational Safety and Health Administration (OSHA) A federal agency created to save lives, prevent injuries, and protect the health of America's workers.

onlay A dental restoration that covers the entire chewing surface, plus at least one or more tooth cusps. Usually used for back teeth.

organic mercury   The most toxic form of mercury, organic mercury occurs in carbon-based compounds and exemplifies the chemical meaning of organic, which is "compounds that are carbon-based."

peptides   A very small protein, comprised of less than 50 amino acids. Glutathione is a peptide.

periodontal disease   An infection of the gums, periodontal ligament and bone that surround and support the teeth.

pervasive developmental disorders (PDD)   Five disorders, all of which show, to varying degrees, repetitive patterns, poor social interactions, and delays in developing normal communication skills. Autism is one of the five.

poison   A substance that is usually very unstable and is harmful or fatal when introduced into the body.

porcelain-to-metal crowns   A dental restoration where a porcelain material is baked to an underlying metal dental crown.

pro-amalgam dentists   Dentists who support and promote the use of mercury amalgam (silver) fillings.

psychosomatic symptoms   Symptoms that are believed to result from thought processes and emotions rather than from an actual physical cause.

Rett Syndrome   A serious learning and developmental disorder. One of the five pervasive developmental disorders (PDD).

Rubin, Paul   A prominent Seattle mercury free and safe dentist and one of the original members of the IAOMT. He is also active in educating the public about the health hazards of fluoride.

rubber dam   A thin square of latex or silicone rubber whose function is to isolate the tooth/teeth being treated from its environment, in particular from saliva and bacteria in the oral cavity.

safe amalgam removal protocol   The procedure a mercury safe dentist follows when removing mercury amalgam fillings, to minimize a patient's exposure to mercury.

St. Francis Academy   The first dental school in the U.S. Founded in Baltimore, Maryland in 1828, and renamed the Baltimore College of Dental Surgery in 1839.

Stejskal, Vera   The inventor of the Melisa® test and one of the founders of MELISA Medica Foundation, an organization that promotes research on metal allergy and treatments

sulfhydryl group   A compound that contains a functional group composed of a sulfur atom and a hydrogen atom (-SH).

Taveau, Auguste   The Frenchman who created mercury amalgam fillings in 1816 by mixing elemental mercury with filings from silver coins.

teratogenic substance   Any substance that disrupts the growth and development of the embryo and fetus, leading to neurological and central nervous system disorders.

thimerosal   A mercury-based compound used in vaccinations as a preservative. Although it's being phased out, it's still found in vaccinations today. Each vaccination preserved with thimerosal can contain as much as 237 mcg of mercury. One mcg of mercury contains about 4 trillion atoms of mercury.

time-weighted average (TWA)   The average amount of a substance considered "safe" to be exposed to over a workday of a specified length of time, typically eight to 10 hours.

tolerance testing   A method of testing an individual's response to a vitamin or nutritional supplement.

tooth grinding   The process of grinding the teeth of the upper and lower jaw together during sleep or naps. Also referred to as "bruxism."

toxic   Relating to or caused by a poison or toxin.

toxin   A poisonous substance that is usually very unstable and is notably toxic when introduced into the body.

urine mercury challenge test   This test requires a pharmaceutical chelator that aggressively seeks out mercury throughout the body, but not in the brain or central nervous system (CNS).

urine mercury unprovoked test   This urine test records the amount of mercury the body naturally removes via the kidneys. No chelator is used.

Urine Porphyrin Profile   A non-invasive test that can detect a recent exposure to mercury.

vitamin C infusions   Providing a patient with vitamin C intravenously, also referred to as an IV drip.

World Health Organization (WHO)   The directing and coordinating authority on international health issues. The WHO "strives to bring the highest level of health to all peoples" and guarantees that employees are protected against both clinically significant symptoms and nonspecific symptoms.

Index

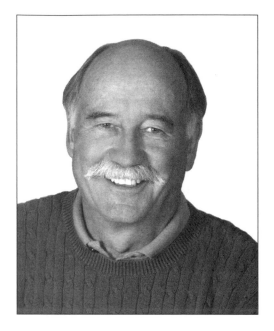

Dr. Tom McGuire has been a mercury free, holistic dentist for over 30 years and is an innovator and leader in holistic dental wellness. He is considered to be one of the world's leading authorities on the effects of mercury amalgam (silver) fillings on overall health, chronic mercury poisoning, and mercury detoxification.

In 2004 Dr. Tom formed the International Association of Mercury Free Dentists (IAMFD) to provide a more effective way for patients to find mercury free and mercury safe dentists. In 1997 he founded the Dental Wellness Institute with the goal of bridging the gap between the dental and medical profession. He has authored a number of books, including the bestselling *Tooth Trip* and *Tooth Fitness*. His most recent book, *Mercury Detoxification*, is the definitive book on how to safely remove mercury from the body.

Dr. Tom's books have also been published in Great Britain, Canada, and the Netherlands. He has appeared on national television, and has been featured in many popular magazines, including *Newsweek, Time, Esquire, Reader's Digest, The Christian Science Monitor*, and *Prevention Magazine*, to name a few. In addition, Rodale Press and Psychology Today carried the *Tooth Trip* in their book clubs, and his books have been Book-of-the-Month Club feature selections.

Visit Dr. Tom on his website, www.dentalwellness4u.com.

He resides in Sebastopol, California, with his wife Zoe.